Symbiotic Safety

Safety and Operations Work Better Together

John Brattlof &
Todd C. Smith

AUSTIN
BROTHERS PUBLISHING

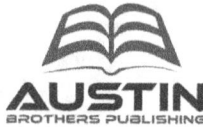

Symbiotic Safety: Safety and Operations Work Better
Together
© 2020 by John Brattlof and Todd Smith
Published by Austin Brothers Publishing

ISBN: 978-1-7333130-9-4
Library of Congress Number: 2020920759

Printed in the United States

Acknowledgments

We want to thank several colleagues and safety professionals listed below who directly or indirectly contributed to this project and the team at Austin Brothers Publishing. Without the effort, passion, and commitment of many safety professionals whose ideas and experiences have impacted our lives as construction safety professionals, we would not have been able to write this book. The lessons we have learned throughout our careers we wish to share to inspire construction veterans still battling in the field and rookies just starting to find their way on the path to a career in construction safety.

- **Richard E. Slater**, Owner, CEO, Slater Painting
- **Steve Burch**, COO, White Construction Company
- **Pat Walsh**, CSP, Walsh Safety Consulting LLC
- **J. Eric Stefan**, CSHO, Safe Construction Consulting LLC
- **Rick Segura**, Senior Safety Manager, Vaughn Construction, Harvey Cleary Builders
- **Mark Gaskamp**, CSP, Senior Vice President, Marsh Wortham Insurance Company
- **Bennett Ghormley**, Co-Founder, Zero Injury Institute
- **Dr. E. Scott Geller**, Virginia Tech, Director, Center of Applied Behavior Systems
- **Bill Sims, Jr.**, President, The Bill Sims Company
- **Joann Natarajan**, Compliance Assistance Specialist, OSHA, Austin Area

Contents

Preface

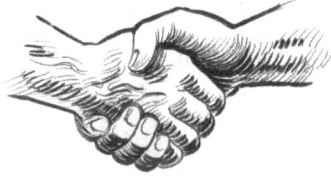

Safety programs have been evolving and adapting for many years. The variety of approaches to safety can be diverse, ranging from extreme micromanagement of every task to a hands-off approach with minimal involvement. This range is sometimes incorrectly assumed as the level of commitment an organization has toward safety. Safety commitment should not be measured by how much resources are invested in safety activities. Rather, safety activities should be so integrated into the normal operations of an organization that there appears to be very little *safety activity*.

Safety and operations can work together to make the organization safe and efficient. This symbiotic relationship helps an organization achieve operational excellence and safety excellence without developing competing priorities. This symbiotic relationship is not easy to achieve. To prevent operations from neglecting safety, the modern safety professional must be an extraordinary leader.

We published *Symbiotic Safety* because we believe that construction safety professionals are extraordinary people, doing extraordinary things under extraordinary circumstances. Rarely in a for-profit environment could one find a group of passionate, dedicated professionals, from such varying backgrounds, all directly working together on a virtual team for a single humanitarian purpose. Perhaps you might say this is a bit lofty for construction safety. Fair enough, but we are indeed a unique lot. This group of individuals is uniquely placed in a highly competitive world.

The construction industry still contributes something tangible, visible, and real to society — we build things. There was nothing, and now there is a building. How did that happen? Real people creating tangible, touchable things. How do you go from a hole in the ground to that beautiful, glass, 34 story box? How do you do this safely? I know this is a bit old fashioned. Safety Knowledge, Safety Ideas, Safety Programs do not compete from one construction company to the next. Whether it is general contractors, subcontractors, concrete, electrical, or painting, we do not have proprietary safety information. You will never hear "I'm sorry, but that is our Fall Protection Program. I really can't discuss how we keep our workers from dying from falls on our job sites. We do not want to lose our competitive advantage in the safety market."

Our Safety Programs, our Best Practices, our Lessons Learned (both the good ones and the bad ones), these are all willingly shared with our safety professional colleagues. Just say you're in the Construction Safety Professional Club, and there is no special handshake or secret codeword needed, you are in. What do you need? How can I help? What problem are you trying to solve? This is a typical response when one safety professional seeks out another when confronted with a safety challenge. No mystery here; where else do you find a group of unrelated people dedicated to the noble mission of keeping people safe from injury in a dynamic industry where fatalities and serious injury are a daily reality?

Safety professionals can provide real value to an organization. Not just perceived value, or an assumption that costs are being reduced via fewer accidents. Safety should never be reduced to a cost-benefit evaluation. Instead, the modern safety professional will seek to use safety and operations equally to make both results improve.

Chapter 1

The Symbiotic Relationship

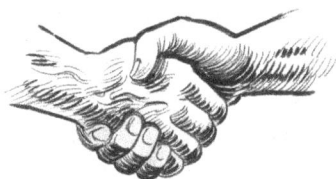

In many organizations, there has been a struggle between safety and operations. While acknowledging that safety is important, operations pays the bills, keeps the lights on, and pays the salaries. Safety is often perceived as a necessary evil. No one wants to see people hurt, so it is hard to argue against safety programs.

In the past few decades, safety professionals have done such a great job promoting the value of safety that is given a modicum of support by operations personnel. It's not that they have all bought into and understand the value of safety; they have just been conditioned to know that fighting safety rarely turns out well for them. It has become akin to paying taxes. I wouldn't say I like to pay that money, and I guess there is a benefit to us all. But I just don't want to face the consequences of getting caught not paying the taxes due.

What if safety was not loved as much as taxes? Can modern safety professionals use safety to make the entire organization better? What if safety programs improved productivity? Quality? Costs? And not just in theory but with definable, quantifiable, and tangible results? It is possible. To do so, the modern safety professional has to make some fundamental shifts in the way safety is executed within the organization.

Twenty years ago, I transitioned from petro-chemical construction to commercial construction. Both are still construction, but the differences were profound. Few commercial owners value safety even remotely as much as petro-chemical owners do. The number of details to manage in a large commercial project is mind-boggling. Twenty years later, I am still amazed at how so many moving parts and pieces can be brought together to create a commercial building.

Even with the incredible amount of details, the other vast difference was the lack of clear procedures. It seemed that commercial construction was too complex to be done systemically. Instead of a finely choreographed system for completing each step, it looked more like a forest fire in which each day assessed the most pressing needs, and attention was given to the most pressing problem of the day. The project leaders worked as hard as possible each day and did not know there was a better way. There were very detailed schedules created for every task required to build the building. But on many occasions, I heard a Project Superintendent tell me that those colorful charts and graphs are nice, but they don't get a building built. It did not take long before I realized that this process seemed to work for the first 75% of the project, but once the end was in sight, the lack of planning almost always slammed right into the reality of the final completion date. Then panic mode kicked in, and safety suffered greatly.

Takeaway 1: Focus on the process, not just the outcome.

"Focus on the process, not the outcome," – Nick Saban.

One of the most impressive things about watching Nick Saban coach is when the team is celebrating a touchdown, and yet he is fuming mad. With the level of talent that Alabama recruits, many times, the play can break down, and physical talent can make good things happen. Most coaches would be happy for the outcome, But not Nick Saban. This focus on the process and not the results is why he won five National Championships in an eight-year stretch at Alabama.

Most safety professionals are focused on safety outcomes. Examples include accident/incident rates, EMR, near misses, violations noted on safety audits. Some even include leading indicators such as JSA's completed, training attendance, safety toolbox talks delivered, etc. But very few safety professionals bother to get involved in the operational facets of the project.

As I started my safety visits to each project, one of the first questions became, "How is the schedule?" It is obvious that when there were operational struggles, safety on the project would also suffer. In the fire fighting mode, you tackle the most pressing problems first. If there has not been an uncomfortable amount of accidents, then the schedule gets all priority. Also, in fire fighting mode, there is very little true planning as to what will be happening several weeks from now. Once the fire fighting mode kicks in, it is incredibly difficult to get out of that mode.

Takeaway 2: Operational failures lead to safety failures.

When we arrived at the job site to start our work, something had changed. We observed that all of the ductwork had been installed, blocking our access to paint the ceiling above the ducts and the walls behind it? (At the Pre-Con meeting, in the trailer, it was never mentioned that all the ductwork would be installed before we started painting.) We quickly went to the job trailer to speak to the GC Superintendent about this *little problem.*

We were told that the owner had delayed the contract and funding for the painting and that the HVAC contract was already funded. Additionally, the HVAC sub had adequate manpower to install the ductwork per the schedule, and they could not promise that manpower later if they could not install immediately. So they installed it.

After some heated back and forth between Project Managers, our Superintendent asked the GC Superintendent, "How are we supposed to paint above and behind the duct? The lift can't reach it, and the scaffold can't reach it. The only way we can paint it is if you take down the ducts."

He responded, "Well, that's not going to happen. Do what you gotta do. Just get it done."

When there are operational failures, it almost always put stress on the safety of the project. Many construction firms may have the fortitude not to let safety slip in these type situations, but it does take a toll on safety either way. Safety professionals do not get more credibility by being able to stop work. They may get enough support from upper management, but they are still perceived as the cause of the problem. Savvy safety professionals may push back to make sure the real point of failure is known, but that leads to finger-pointing and a sense of us versus them. The modern safety professional will understand that when operations fails, safety is not far behind.

Takeaway 3: Safety professionals can become too focused on safety metrics alone.

Unfortunately, many safety professionals do not fully grasp the operational impact on safety. When the safety professional is only focused on the results of Safety Audits, training, JSA's, accident rates, etc., they ignore the dramatic impact that operations has on safety performance. The modern safety professional should be interested in safety, but also the affects schedule, budget, and quality have on the project. All of these factors work together to create the success or failure of a project.

One common cause of this myopic view of safety is allowing the safety functions to stand apart from the operations functions. For instance, a stand-alone Safety Manual creates the impression that there are operational procedures and then safety procedures. In every case possible, the safety concerns should be integrated into the Operations Manual. There should not be procedures that explain how to operate productively and then another set of procedures to operate safely. There should be one set of procedures that lead to safe, productive, quality, cost-effective work.

Safety training programs should not be solely focused on safety rules but should instead focus on helping employees be excellent workers in all facets of the job. Since safety training is much more common and easily accessible, therefore, the modern safety professional could also use that time to get operational experts to help train employees of more productive ways to accomplish the work or how to achieve better quality. These training venues are always well received by employees as they feel they are learning a skill, not just a set of rules.

In the example above, the GC staff did the best they knew how to do with what they had. With a great desire to accommodate the owner, they allowed the sequencing to become unmanageable. They allowed the duct work to get installed in a way that made it impossible to paint safely. When safety professionals are focused solely on safety metrics, it would never occur to them to promote the concepts of proper sequencing and instruct on the hazards associated with improper sequencing during their safety training. Focusing on the safety rules alone does not help the modern safety professional address all sources of safety hazards within the operations of a construction firm.

Takeaway 1: Focus on the process, not just the outcome.

Takeaway 2: Operational failures lead to safety failures.

Takeaway 3: Safety professionals can become too focused on safety metrics alone.

Chapter 2

Safety Excellence is Dependent on Operational Excellence

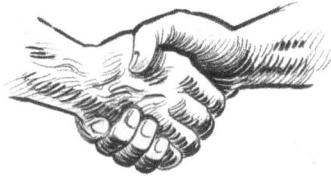

James is a great carpenter. He worked in the maintenance shop for many years with me. One of his common tasks was to build out portable office trailers for new projects. He had been doing this for years and always finished on time with a true craftsman level of quality. James was a great employee. He produced great work and never created any problems. That is until his supervisor started hounding him about safety.

Adam had been the maintenance supervisor for decades. His department was productive and did not have any injuries for decades. Since the company was always talking about safety at every possible opportunity, Adam thought he should as well.

James was ripping long sheets of plywood on a table saw when Adam walked by. Wanting to promote safety, Adam assessed the situation and saw that James was not wearing any gloves.

"Get your gloves on, James!" Adam yelled over the noise of the saw.

James finished the cut and found some gloves to wear. Adam thought he had performed his role as a supervisor extremely well and went about his day pleased with himself. This safety stuff isn't so hard.

Later that day, the ambulance arrived to take James, and his severed thumb tip, to the ER. Gloves do not protect a hand from table saw hazards. James had been ripping plywood so long on that saw that he did not even realize how he had been doing it. For decades, James had been guiding the wood with his right hand until his hand hit the guard, and he would pull away. The work gloves made sure he did not feel the guard, and his thumb went right into the spinning blade. The first day of trying to be safe resulted in his first injury.

Takeaway 1: Creating safety excellence must include operational excellence.

Safety professionals have become myopic in their views of what makes an organization successful. Unless you work for the National Safety Council, your employer is not in business to make people safer. Your company exists to provide the marketplace goods or services that the marketplace is willing to pay for. Safety programs are usually implemented to decrease the cost of unwanted accidents or for a moral obligation to reduce the pain and suffering of employees. Many organizations will claim both are valid reasons. Too often, the safety professional forgets the main goal of the company and focuses on just reducing accidents.

To be truly successful, the safety professional needs to be aware that operational excellence creates safety excellence. When operations are running smoothly, there are fewer variables present. Fewer variables lead to fewer opportunities for unplanned events. Safety programs should not compete with operational efforts.

Adam never attempted to help James do his job better. He never examined how the work was being done and if there were ways to improve the operation. Adam simply knew he was supposed to support safety, so he thought making James wear gloves would show that safety was important. By itself, this was not a bad thing, but without attempting to improve the entire process, Adam just made things worse.

Takeaway 2: Operational excellence cannot solely focus on production metrics.

When asked, "what does operational excellence look like," most people will use production metrics to quantify results. Increased production rates over the short term do not define operational excellence. To achieve operational excellence, four categories of metrics must excel: Safety, Quality, Productivity, and Cost. These are fundamentals that anyone in business understands.

There will be some within the organization that will use cost metrics to define operational excellence. Cost is extremely important. If the price point of your goods or services is above the market rates, you will create an incredible product that no one buys. By definition, that is worthless. Even worse, you sell a product that costs more to make than the proceeds from selling it.

Quality is equally important. If the customer has expectations about the quality of the product that are not met, the customer will go elsewhere. If producing a product that does meet specifications requires multiple attempts and generates excessive waste, the cost becomes prohibitive. In order to achieve operational excellence, the product must be reproduced without flaw or waste. The level of importance in quality varies by market. If building a large museum or computer chip manufacturing facility, quality is extremely important. When building a low rent apartment complex, quality becomes much less important.

Safety is the oddball in the group. Does the customer care about the safety program of the provider of goods and services? In markets where the vendor's safety performance will directly impact the customer (such as a chemical plant), safety will matter to the customer. In most business operations, the customer does not care about how safely the product is made. Most safety professionals bristled at that statement. So, look at the label of the shirt you are wearing. Was it made in a country that is known to have strict labor and safety regulations enforced? What about the chair you are sitting in while reading this book? To the customer, price and quality are the two main factors in making purchases.

Operational excellence is created when all aspects of the production of your product or service operate without waste. No waste of time, personnel, product, or money is acceptable.

Takeaway 3: A safety professional must be just as concerned about quality, productivity, and cost, and other sectors should focus on safety.

Safety professionals should strive to be operational experts as well. When safety professionals advocate for safety without regard for the other fundamentally important aspects of the organization, they begin to lose credibility. Operations personnel see safety as a necessary liability and not as an important asset. Being perceived as only a cost or hindrance to getting work done does not help the safety professional become effective. When a safety professional invests time and energy to understand and improve the complete operation of the organization truly, then he can be perceived as an asset that is here to make things better, not worse. How can anyone make a process safer if they do not fully understand the entire process?

Instead of Adam giving a token effort to find some way to bring safety concerns to James, maybe the accident would not have happened. Adam could have spent some time to discover how James built out the office trailers. He could have discovered any planning in place to reduce the number of cuts needed or the amount of time walking back and forth measuring. Symbiotic Safety could be developed if the safety professional understood that reducing material handling and the number of cuts needed would help both the cost, time, and risk of the process.

It is disingenuous to expect operations to actively participate in safety if safety professionals will not actively participate in operations. You may have a friend or coworker who is always asking you for favors but never offers anything in return. You know, the person you avoid at work. Many times, safety professionals become that person to operations workers. Always asking to add more requirements and tasks in the name of safety. If it is true that safety should be everyone's responsibility, then why is that not true for other critical aspects of the organization. Why are safety professionals not expected to find ways to make the operation more cost-effective or productive? To get productive buy-in from all areas of operations toward enacting safety procedures, the safety professional must also understand and consider the other critical areas as well. safety professionals should seek complete organizational support.

Takeaway 4: Creating safety excellence must include operational excellence.

Takeaway 5: Operational excellence cannot solely focus on production metrics.

Takeaway 6: A safety professional must be just as concerned about quality, productivity, and cost as those sectors should focus on safety.

Chapter 3

The Cost-Benefit Illusion of Safety

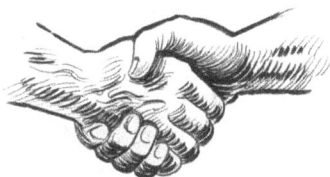

My First Safety Rodeo: Lessons Learned

The 82nd Airborne Division of the US Army taught me many things, among them "Never jump the chain of command," "Fifteen minutes early is on time, five minutes early is late and later than that is not an option," and "Clean, dry socks are precious in the field."

Another lesson comes to mind, "Training, Training, Training, if ain't raining, we ain't training." It seemed like it was always raining in Fort Bragg, North Carolina, and it seemed like we were always training, especially Combat Task Training. Fifty tasks related to combat, broken down by steps, and the participants had to demonstrate proficiency in the task to receive a "GO." This was a GO/NO GO process, and if the soldier did not meet the standard, he/she would perform it again and again until minimal mastery was achieved.

We would take five of these tasks at a time in our platoon and have a *Safety Rodeo* during our scheduled training time. Training stations were led by NCOs (Non-Commissioned Officers, Sergeants to non-military folks), and each group would move from station to station about every 45 minutes. First Aid, Rifle Maintenance, etc. soldiers could never be too good at these tasks, and I was amazed at how effective this technique was. A sense of pride in accomplishment was instilled, friendly competition was created, and it was even fun, at times. I try to implement these elements in my approach to safety with my commercial painters.

As a new OSHA Outreach Construction Safety trainer and a Safety Guy, I started my Safety Director position with the knowledge that my workers were severely under-trained. It was simply not a function of a small to medium-sized construction company to spend time and money on safety training in the relatively safe field of commercial painting. But I was determined to improve my fledgling safety program and pitch my boss on the idea of a Safety Rodeo.

I prepared my presentation and confidently entered my boss' office armed with the concept of the five training stations I would include in our first annual Safety Rodeo; 40-minute rotations, and a list of five takeaways from each station and we would use volunteer trainers from other trades and GCs to deliver the training for our morning long safety training event. I selected training in areas that were challenging for us from my job site observations—Ergonomics, Fall Protection, Scaffold Safety, and Ladder Safety. I even included one of our major trade partners, Sherwin Williams, to help train our workers on the safe use of spray-painting equipment.

My boss patiently listened to my enthusiastic delivery, and I could tell he liked the Army's successful model that I referenced and Sherwin Williams being involved. Finally, when I finished, he said, "I like it. How much is this going to cost?"

Well, I hadn't really thought about that part, and he knew it. He nodded and said we could do this as part of a safety training/holiday party for the guys... "I just need a budget."

I felt good about the exchange and told him I would get a budget back to him by the end of the day. I hurried back to my office and calculated my costs for my Safety Rodeo/Holiday Party. Safety equipment, signage, gift cards for the winning group as judged by the trainers, and of course, lunch for 80. It was just over $2,000, and I quickly went back to my boss with my budget. He looked at it and then back at me, "What about the cost of paying 80 guys for 8 hours? I assume that they will not be going back to work after this."

"No," I mumbled as he started rattling off numbers as he described each to me as he entered them into his calculator. "Eighty employees, average $16 per hour, 8 hours" as he tore off the tape and handed it to me... "that's about $10,000."

An awkward silence fell upon the room...How had I missed that? Then he asked me, "What will I be getting for my $12,000?"

Was this a rhetorical question, I thought. Somehow, I managed to respond, "Safety training, improved morale, and fewer injuries."

Fortunately, I was allowed to proceed with my first construction Safety Rodeo, and it was a success. I was surprised my boss had supported me after I missed 80 percent of the costs. But the workers were trained, safety was given its due, and the first annual Safety Rodeo has continued for ten years. In fact, I was able to create a Safety Rodeo for nearly 200 workers with the OSHA Partnership with Associated Builders and Contractors-Central Texas Chapter. It's also still going strong after seven years.

I don't know if that first Rodeo had returned $12,000 worth of benefit the following year. But we did start our new safety culture, and I learned valuable lessons: Costs always matter, return on investment always matters, and a successful safety culture starts with trust between the owner and the safety guy.

Takeaway 1: Quantifying the real cost of safety is difficult.

The most frequently overlooked area of safety is the actual cost of implementing safety programs. Safety equipment is a real expense. Soon it wears out, and more equipment is needed. Someone must research which equipment is needed, identify the best manufacturer, where to purchase the equipment with the best terms, how the equipment will be distributed, where the equipment will be stored, how will replacements be provided, and who will oversee all of this. All of these are expenses above simply looking at the purchase cost per item.

The CFO of a construction company endeavored to quantify what it took for the accounting department to process one invoice. From the perspective of the safety professional, this means determining a job number and maybe a cost code. But then what happens? My CFO friend explained the long and arduous process of getting invoices approved, coded, input into a cost system, having a check cut, balancing the checkbook, developing financial reports, and tax reports. Their analysis showed it cost the company $173 to process each invoice. Few safety professionals consider this cost in determining the value of a purchase.

Safety training takes time, and time is money. As I learned from attempting to plan a safety training rodeo, most employees are paid while trained. Other programs take time, as well. A 15-minute stretch and flex program in the morning does not seem to be a heavy cost. If the project is working any overtime, this time is quantified as time and a half. A project with 100 workers and a composite rate of $20/hour will spend $750 each day to start a stretch and flex program ($20 * 1.5 * 100 * .25). On an 18-month job, this program would add $292,500 just to have a 15-minute stretch and flex program to start each day.

Some costs are not easily quantifiable. Logically, if a worker or supervisor is focused on a safety task, they cannot be focused on other tasks. Every moment focused on safety will take the focus off something else.

Is safety worth the cost? Of course! Few safety professionals are trained to fully appreciate the scope and implications of all costs associated with safety programs and equipment.

Takeaway 2: Quantifying the actual savings of safety is impossible.

Occasionally evidence of training's return on investment can be demonstrated. One of my stations at the Safety Rodeo was Ergonomics, more specifically proper lifting technique training. I included this class because we had a string of back injuries mostly from older workers, primarily foreman, lifting machines, equipment, or materials, and ended up straining their back. The lift training, conducted by our insurance guy who was a CSP, specifically used the same items we lifted on the job to conduct his training. We included this station each year, and believe it or not, we have not had a back injury since.

However, there are too many variables in construction to predict the real savings created by safety programs accurately. There is no doubt that safety can reduce risk and lower the chances or severity of accidents. Unless an organization is able to run double blind concurrent experiments, the savings is theoretical. Historical data can show reductions in accident frequency and severity due to safety programs. The Hawthorne Studies during the great depression (1927–1932) showed that just giving attention to people and their processes had short term benefits to production. This makes the safety professional wrestle with the dilemma: did the safety program cause the positive effect, or did shining the spotlight on the people and process create the positive effect? Variables in the science of chance and psychology make accurate savings quantification extremely difficult.

Takeaway 3: Accidents happen within great safety programs.

Early in a large industrial construction project, the project realized a milestone goal of 500,000 manhours without a recordable accident of any kind. To celebrate this achievement, a catered lunch was provided, along with a short ceremony, and some thank you gifts for the workers. Small pocketknives were purchased with the company name and 500,000 manhours accident-free printed on each. The lunch and ceremony were perfect. Management was extremely proud of the safety milestone (which by then was over 700,000 manhours without any recordable injuries). The workers certainly liked the free BBQ and had a sense of pride in being recognized for their hard work.

Within one hour of the celebration, a group of workers was walking back to their work area. One of the men noticed a bunch of extra threads sticking out of the back pocket of the fire-retardant coveralls of the man walking in front of him. In an attempt to be helpful (and use his new safety knife), he grabbed the bundle of threads and attempted to cut it off for his friend. Not knowing what was happening behind him, the man swiped his hand to knock off whatever was pulling on his coveralls. In less than an hour after the celebration, the site had its first recordable hand laceration! In an attempt to celebrate safety success, they provided the mechanism for the first injury.

A safety professional once had a recordable injury requiring surgery for trying to put a new 5-gallon water bottle on the water cooler. A subcontractor was having difficulty getting work due to an EMR of 1.77. They had zero accidents related to their work, but four workers in one truck were rear-ended while their truck was waiting at a red light. A very safe worker can miss the last step of a ladder and hyperextend his knee, causing a large claim. Great safety programs can only reduce the chances, never eliminate accidents.

The Safety Rodeo allowed me to focus our training stations on the areas that we incurred the most injuries. While our training was conducted by exceptional trainers and specifically focused on preventing ladders, falls, and lifting related injuries, to this day, these remain the areas where we have our most recordable injuries. Over the past three years, the last five accidents we had were fall from a ladder, trip on floor, fall from scaffold, fall from climbing down from an aerial lift, and fall from ladder.

Takeaway 7: Quantifying the real cost of safety is difficult.

Takeaway 8: Quantifying the actual savings of safety is impossible.

Takeaway 9: Accidents happen within great safety programs.

Chapter 4

Compliance Based Programs Defeat Great Safety Results

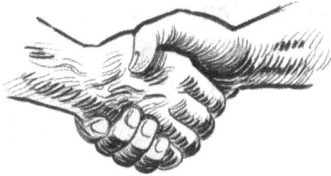

Have you ever had those moments when you see something and cannot accurately process what you see? Your eyes tell a story, but you cannot make any sense of it, so you freeze and stare until something, anything, makes sense.

Many years ago, I was a Safety Supervisor on a large industrial project in west Texas. The contractor was extremely invested in safety. There were numerous full-time safety professionals assigned to the project. Every training, motivational, and monitoring program you could think of was used. There was a zero-tolerance policy for safety violators. If you complied with the rules, you could get paid handsomely; if you broke the rules, immediate termination. This company put its money where its mouth is regarding safety.

That is why I froze when I saw the painter that day. He was in an awkward position, trying to touch up paint on the outside of a very tall vessel. He was standing on an array of pipes and reaching up to paint some new conduit that had been added to the side of the vessel. All of this was about 90 feet above the ground. This painter knew that if he did not comply with the 100% tie-off rule, he would be fired. So he had a harness on with his lanyard attached to something.

That something is what I could not believe. This man had wrapped his lanyard around three small diameter conduits that came out of the vessel for about 18 inches, turned a 90, and went down, vertically 75 feet. Three times before I could get high enough to get his attention without startling him, I saw the lanyard loop slip over the elbow joint and fall down the conduit. Three times I saw the painter grab the lanyard and put it back on the horizontal stub.

After getting the painter into a safe position, we started a heated discussion. Both of us were dumbfounded at the ignorance of the other. I could not believe he had put himself at such great risk, and he could not believe I was threatening his job. He was convinced that since he was tied off, he had broken no rules. As I tried to explain that his tie-off point was woefully inadequate, he just kept insisting that he did nothing wrong and was tied off the entire time. Somehow, following the rules became the goal, and being safe was not considered.

Takeaway 1: Compliance is only a strategy of safe job sites.

Sometimes we tend to forget that our perception of being in compliance with CFR 1926 does not ensure that we have a safe workplace. We ask ourselves, is this activity in compliance? At any level of the organization/ team (Owner, Project Manager, Safety Director, Superintendent, Foreman, Trade Worker), we can manipulate and interpret the construction safety standards to say, "Yes, we are in compliance. We are safe."

Our painter in this story demonstrates the complacency that accident-free work generates and how we can be conditioned to believe we are safe. Other levels of the team must be able to critically assess daily activities and ask, "How can we be safer? Is this the safest way to perform this work?" Compliance is not wrong; it is merely part of the big picture. When we sacrifice the big picture for the small picture, safety can be compromised

When we perform a job site inspection, we ask, "Is there good hazard control?" When we conduct an OSHA Partnership job site monthly safety report, the categories for reporting our job site inspections are Fall Hazards, Electrical Hazards, Struck By Hazards, Caught in Between Hazards, and Other Hazards. Are these metrics an effective way to measure safety and mitigate risk?

When we review the performance of a Safety Director, Safety Program, are we working safely? What about an OSHA 300 Form when we have few accidents or no OSHA recordable incidents, are we working safely? When there are more accidents and more OSHA recordable incidents from one year as compared to the last, are we not as safe as the previous year? Is the Safety Director great one year and then someone to blame the following year because the trend of the metrics in a negative direction?

A company safety strategy must determine how organizational resources, skills, and competencies should be combined to generate the best possible results. This means developing team strategies within a company. Each team should have its own strategy to ensure that its day-to-day activities make safety part of every decision.

A commercial construction company's team strategies must lead directly to the achievement of organizational strategy. All levels of strategy support and enhance each other to ensure optimal job site safety. When an owner wants to have zero accidents, when a Project Manager wants no lost time injury costs on his job, when the Superintendent wants to be efficient with his time and not have to manage injuries, or when a worker is trying to finish a task as quickly as possible without becoming injured… is it a strategy or a goal? Literally and figuratively, our team has to provide a safety net for other levels. Compliance helps us to build this net.

While compliance is a reasonable strategy to improve job site safety, it is not a goal. Compliance limits the potential of a safety culture as compared to a best practice-based culture that promotes worker engagement. Goals have to be SMART: Specific, Measurable, Attainable, Relevant, Time-based. A Compliance-only Strategy is just not smart.

Takeaway 2: Strategies are not the goal.

The goal is for every worker to participate actively in safety. True engagement and safety awareness is the result of a dynamic safety culture. Dr. E. Scott Geller, an expert in human behavior, says that Proactively Caring for People (PC4P) is the goal. Workplace safety and identifying human factors can reduce accidents, incidents, minimize risks in the workplace, and improve overall performance. For example, encouraging conversation in the workplace, educating, and enable champions from across the workforce to support keeping people safe, accepting education and training provided by peers.

When the painter was confronted about his tie-off point, a heated but productive conversation resulted. When a worker believes that he knows how to perform their work safely and it is hazardous, this is a critical and teachable moment. If the safety professional writes up the worker for a safety violation, sends him home, or even terminates his position, this action is counterproductive and weakens the safety culture. What will his takeaway from this experience be?

The goal is raising awareness of safety by building relationships within the team and working together to accomplish a best practice-driven safety culture. How can a safety culture grow if, at a critical moment, when a worker could be taught, he is summarily punished? What will he say to his coworkers, "I tried to follow the rules and be safe and look what I got for it."

Relationship building allows safety professionals to gain access to worker trust. Trust is essential to enhance the strategy of safety compliance.

Takeaway 3: Focus on compliance limits focus on accident prevention.

When we focus on compliance, we miss the opportunity to emphasize a worker's role in controlling hazards. We can identify the most hazardous tasks in a vacuum based on our history and OSHA 300 and then list their corresponding remediation on a Job Hazard

Analysis. However, performing the actual tasks must address multiple variables that lead to injuries.

How can we account for distractions, heat, fatigue, standing water, mindset, other trades working in close quarters, debris, meeting deadlines, or human error? Compliance focuses on risks that have been associated with tasks. These are truly trailing indicators. Accident prevention requires more than just explaining a rule to a worker and threatening them if they violate it. Accident prevention requires experience, judgment, and anticipation.

How can we empower our workers to assess risks on the fly and ask them to make the best decision possible? We can ask this because they have done this many times before. They need to use their experience and safety knowledge not only for their benefit but for new employees and the rest of the company. If the safety professional initiates a dialogue to review the hazards, it needs to be a free flow exchange of information. Show the worker you care, explain the why and how of potential accident causation, and encourage and thank the worker for performing the work safely.

A company's safety culture must be dynamic, using compliance as a starting point, but tapping into work insights and advice requires a level of confidence in employees that is demonstrated daily. Saying "We care about our worker's safety" on a t-shirt company stationary is a nice thought, but are we utilizing the best resource to improve job site safety, senior worker experience?

A *Compliance Mentality* means safety is only as good as the effectiveness of enforcing the rules. Do you always receive a ticket when you speed? Do you ever try a strawberry when you are shopping at HEB? Do you declare every dollar you earn to the IRS? We always think we are right, and no matter how nicely we are told otherwise when we are told we are wrong, we don't like it. Many times when a worker is confronted for being *out of compliance*, he is thinking this, "Why me? Other people are doing the same thing." Or "Ok, I am not wearing my glasses, but that guy is standing on the railing of the scissor lift."

Let us not underestimate our workers' intelligence, creativity, and ingenuity. They have performed work without accidents many times before, and all have instinctive self-preservation instincts. They can understand the why and the how of safety. As safety professionals, it is incumbent upon us to have patience and invest time building a relationship with every worker. Not doing so risks that ever-popular "safety, only when the safety guy is on site." The ultimate test of a safety culture is what happens after the safety inspection or when no safety professional is on site.

Takeaway 10: Compliance is only a strategy of safe workplaces.

Takeaway 11: Strategies are not the goal.

Takeaway 12: Focus on compliance limits focus on accident prevention-avoiding hazards if possible, being aware of the highest risk activities.

Chapter 5

How Decisions are made

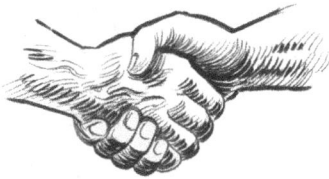

I had no idea why I was sitting in the Cover 3 restaurant with our President, waiting to have lunch with someone from a general contractor. After a short while, I was introduced to the Safety Director from one of our clients, and I still was in the dark about the purpose of our meeting. When we had finished ordering, my boss said, "So I was just wondering, what do we have to do to get more work from you guys? We used to get lots of jobs from you, and it seems like lately, they are few and far between."

The Safety Director leaned forward and said, "Well, things have changed. The projects we are getting are bigger than in the past, and they have more safety requirements. You do a good job for us, but you don't have much of a safety program."

My boss, not a man known for his willingness to concede control, fired back, "Ok. What do we need to do?"

"First of all, you need a full-time Safety Manager, a training program, and a comprehensive safety program," the Safety Director said.

"This safety guy needs to be bilingual, an OSHA Outreach Trainer, and conduct job site inspections. He needs to train your employees in all areas of safety that affect your work. You need to have a safety program."

My boss looked at me and said, "Congratulations, you're my new safety guy." And then back at the Safety Director, "Ok. Here is my new safety guy, can you help him get where he needs to be?"

When we got back to the office, my boss gave me our boilerplate safety policy and a copy of the GC's safety policy. It was then that I started my five-year safety mission with this Safety Director as my mentor, a former Marine. He would say you should do this and I would do it. That first year I brought him in several times to train my foreman in scaffold, ladder, and fall protection safety. He had a command presence with my workers, and I saw him as a role model.

I became an OSHA Outreach Trainer that year and set the goal of redrafting our safety policy, have annual updates, and provide OHSA training in Spanish for all of our employees. I mention the Spanish part because training in Spanish is not simply translating training from English as most people think. Most Spanish speaking trade workers have not spent time in a classroom for many years and never in a class with technical vocabulary and PowerPoint presentations. Besides, simply presenting safety topics and expecting them to be implemented on job sites was a slow and frustrating process—more the result of *MY* unrealistic expectations and learning about the culture of my employees than anything else. The most important lessons I learned about training in Spanish were the most difficult and time-intensive ones. Relationships take time, and trust is not something workers will give you easily. If you doubt this, just look around and see how many people can deliver effective safety training in Spanish; it is a very short list.

I trained all of my workers in the 10 Hour OSHA Construction Safety Course and our Foreman and Superintendents in the 30 Hour OSHA Safety Course. Even our Project Managers would receive the 10 Hour safety course. This was accomplished in the first year, and then I decided that all new employees would also receive the OSHA 10. While my boss did not like training people who left after seasonal work or for no reason at all, "We're just pissing money away," he would say on his bad days, in future years, many of these employees would return to us, so the investment in training and safety was not wasted after all. This level of trained personnel remains in effect today and is still uncommon amongst Central Texas subcontractors.

The second year of our program featured our first Safety Rodeo rotating station training that is still an annual event. In that same year, I became certified as a CPR/First Aid trainer and trained all office staff and Superintendents. We had an ergonomics expert provide training on proper lifting techniques to reduce the number of back injuries. This annual training is still ongoing, and fortunately, we have not had a back injury for the past seven years, after five back injuries in the previous year.

During the third year, we joined the Central Texas OSHA Partnership, and I became Chairman by the end of that year. Our EMR started going down, our Workers

Comp premium as well, and we even started receiving Safety Awards for our program.

In the fourth and fifth years, we started our mandatory Drug Testing program for new hires and random and annual testing for all employees. We were growing considerably, and the challenges of maintaining all of the components in our safety policy were manageable but endless.

The next five years were a time of fine-tuning. There will never be the excitement of starting a new program, and I have since tried to mentor other safety professionals. The young workers today provide some different challenges. The larger our company grows, it seems like our new contracts are with clients who have more complex safety issues than ever before. A few years back, a million-dollar commercial painting contract was rare. Today it seems like we bid these monthly and even have two-million-dollar jobs on the books. I reflect upon the day of that first lunch and how my boss and mentor trusted and supported me to move our program forward. Through their leadership, mentoring, and decision making, we were able to develop our safety program, receive more work, and expand our client base to include some of the largest general contractors in Central Texas.

Takeaway 1: Honest and open communication leads to better decisions.

My boss is not a reactive decision-maker; his decision-making style could be described as slow and steady. For example, we still use a cardstock time card. Time cards were developed in 1722. Any time someone suggests we use electronic record keeping, like some of our competitors, he says, "I will take that under advisement." When he is asked to make work-related decisions, he may say yes, he rarely says no and often says, "I will take it under advisement." This can mean many things. From a soft no to a permanent non-decision to remind me later. I have learned that this is his effective communication and decision-making strategy. He is being honest, answering the question, and let the person asking know that he is not ready to declare his decision even if it is already made.

When he surprised me the most was when he asked the GC Safety Director at that lunch, "What do we need to do?" Hearing the answer and stating this is my new safety guy to me." This meant the decision was made. The response to his question received an immediate and specific response. His decision was also immediate. This indicates he knew the facts regarding the situation at hand, had already developed an action plan, and selected the person to direct and accomplish the task.

Another example is how he decided to reopen our office after we had moved 95% of staff to work at home during the COVID-19 Stay at Home, Stay Safe campaign. One of the Project Managers refused to work from home, and he calmly listened to him defend his position that COVID-19 was a scam and the biggest government conspiracy ever and then allowed him to work at the office.

In early June, another PM who had grudgingly agreed to leave with the others was constantly nudging my boss on how he couldn't take working around his wife and kids anymore. He missed the interaction with his colleagues and said he was losing control of his projects in the field. When he asked me whether I thought we should come back to the office, I said no. He said, "If he doesn't let us come back next week, I am coming anyway."

The self-imposed isolation of COVID-19 seemed to make everyone communicate more clearly and directly than before the pandemic. Our employees just seemed more compelled to articulate any complaint or concern with great detail, albeit normally from a less than objective perspective. When we all had time to think about wanting the old normal back, we relieved the guilt of previous tongue-biting and spoke more freely. This made me a better listener after lots of practice.

Takeaway 2: Clear expectations lead to success.

By providing me with copies of our existing safety policies and authorizing me to use the GC Safety Director as a resource, I knew his expectations. If he would have leaned back in his executive chair, at his desk, and said, "I think it would be nice to have a safety program, don't you," the result would have been quite different. Using the specific examples of our boilerplate safety policy and the GC's safety policy, I could see a clearer idea of what the deliverable would be. This was a great start and led to a successful outcome. I could see what we had in our policy was different than what was happening in the field. The GC's safety program had many areas that commercial painters do not have to address. Therefore, I was able to focus our new program on what we were actually doing and train employees based on the needs identified during the process of developing our safety program.

Another aspect of clear expectations is when leaders establish a standard and infer and imply that they are confident that their employees can implement this standard. Once again, the COVID-19 scenario provided several opportunities for me to practice developing action plans. Having the entire commercial construction industry and the state, city, and county governments pushing the same CDC protocol, the result was a high standard of safety for COVID-19 protection. While exceptions were still observable, the awareness of wearing face coverings, hand washing, and social distancing gained traction at a remarkable rate. Seeing workers violate these guidelines was still common, but a broad-based emphasis on compliance with the COVID-19 Protocol made it become part of commercial construction safety culture.

I used a carrot-stick strategy to encourage our employees to be vigilant about their COVID-19 safety and overall job site safety. I rarely sent workers home for safety violations and bought several lunches for the entire crew when everyone showed extra effort to comply. I also tried to reel in the outliers/violators by offering extra safety glasses, gloves, or face coverings when they were out of compliance. However, if the stick does not exist, the carrot is always expected and soon becomes less effective with workers. I believe we have to inspect what we expect or safety becomes a watered-down version of a *pretty safe* job site falling victim to the "at least nobody got hurt" mantra rather than "how can we do better, how can we be safer" mantra.

Takeaway 3: Developing and implementing an action plan is the first step.

While this may seem rather obvious, I am surprised how many safety professionals don't seem to have developed an effective Action Plan when attacking a problem. Starting with the facts, the best available resources and information available, sampling successful strategies that others have implemented to achieve positive outcomes, we can generate an idea of the direction we are headed. Granted, there are times when it's ok to proceed with a lack of specific plans. My boss was not aware of all of the details of what I needed to develop, implement, and maintain a safety program. He did not have to be. His plan was based on what has become my philosophy, "I don't know what I want, but I know what I don't want—what I have right now." Many times this is a great starting point and can drive any plan from its inception.

Just the other day, I was on a job site where we had a large crew, about 20 of our painters, and the shop area was messy and unorganized, with equipment and lunch boxes scattered everywhere and the entire area filled with empty water bottles. I took pictures of the shop area and sent them to the Foreman, Superintendent, and Project Manager with no text message, just the pictures. I brought my Foreman to the shop area and asked him, "Is this acceptable?" He began talking about having to control so many workers, the fact that the GC had banned water jugs due to their COVID-19 protocol and so he had to bring water bottles for 20 people every day, and more excuses.

I said, "I am not here to criticize you. We need to do better."

My intention was for the Foreman to say no, this is not acceptable and have him develop a plan to improve and maintain a clean shop area and cleaner job site. If I had done it, it would be much less effective and short-lived. By empowering him to develop a plan and show me the results, I could immediately compliment and encourage him. We would have an expectation of what I wanted and the precedent of him knowing what I don't want. That is what you call a teachable moment.

I said, "You know what the standard is for our shop areas, you just received a high school kid as a new painter helper. Use the new kid, come up with a plan, and let me know what you will be doing to prevent this from happening again."

The next morning my Foreman had sent me three pictures of the same areas that I have sent out the day before. The equipment was organized, the floor was clean, and he said the high school kid would be cleaning at the beginning and end of each day. I replied that it looked great and now just to keep it up. He said he wanted a cooler for the water bottles, a garbage can and bags for the shop, and a lock to chain them to our job box so that other trades would not steal the cooler and garbage can.

Later that morning, I arrived with what he had requested. When I returned a few days later, the shop area was clean, our work areas were cleaner, and I gave him a $100 gift card with the compliment for a job well down. Sometimes, things do go as planned.

Takeaway 13: Honest and open communication leads to better decisions.

Takeaway 14: Clear expectations lead to success.

Takeaway 15: Developing and implementing an action plan is the first step.

Chapter 6

Keeping the Role of the safety professional in Perspective

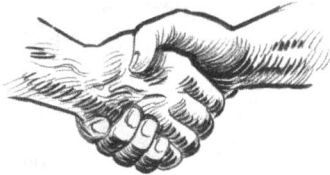

He held the pen in his mouth to sign the Safety Violation Form. I still can't believe I made him do that. But my first official act as a safety professional was to visit an injured worker in the hospital and have him sign our Safety Violation Form with a pen in his mouth.

The Foreman, with five years of experience, who I had recently trained in my OSHA 30 Hour Construction Safety class, was working at a new elementary school that was nearly completed. He and another worker were on-site to complete a punch list and were located on opposite sides of the school. He was on top of a 24-foot ladder in a mechanical room while waiting for the other worker to come and hold the base of his ladder. He described the situation as follows:

"I wanted to get finished and needed to reach a corner to paint it and stepped on the second to the last step. The ladder

lifted up off the floor a couple of inches and set down. Then I stepped on the last step and the ladder lifted up about six inches and set down. Next, I was standing on the end cap of the ladder for just a second and the entire ladder lifted up and I rode it down to the floor. I landed on top of the ladder and could tell both my arms were broken. I had pain in my knee and chin. Blood was coming from my mouth and some of my teeth were loose, one was on the floor. I could not walk and crawled out into the hallway to call for help."

As I was on my way to the hospital in Round Rock, I had heard that he had broken both arms and had pins in one. Three teeth had broken off, and his knee cap was displaced. My mission was to go to the hospital, confirm the details of the incident, and have him sign the safety violation form.

I arrived to find him with both arms suspended in the air by pulleys on a metal frame, his head bandaged, and his wife by his side. After we exchanged some pleasantries, I asked him to tell me what happened. He told me what I referenced above. I asked why the accident happened. He said that he was in a hurry and didn't want to wait for his co-worker (they were almost finished for the day), and he had done it before, and nothing had happened. I thought, "What about the ladder safety rules you violated, not using the last three steps of the ladder, standing on the end cap, having someone hold the base of the extension ladder?" Yet, I said nothing.

I held out my form on a clipboard to have him sign, and he looked at me as if to say, how should I sign? I held the pen up to his mouth, and he scribbled his name. I remember that it was not that different from his normal signature.

Driving home, I felt frustrated and concerned. How could a 30-Hour OSHA trained foreman do this? How could he intentionally violate his training? Was my training to blame? Had I not emphasized ladder safety sufficiently? How could I make him sign with a pen? These questions and more continued to bother me for several days.

I concluded that I never wanted to go and see one of my employees in the hospital again, all of our safety training was going to get better, and everyone will be immediately retrained in ladder safety. This was my fault. We could do better.

With advice from my insurance guy, I spent the next three months actively managing my Foreman's recovery and return to work. I learned about occupational therapy, workers comp, and injury management. Some care providers were more receptive to my presence at his appointments than others, but I always insisted this was a Workers Comp injury, and I am the employer. It helped that I was also a Spanish translator. I brought him to every appointment; follow-ups, dental, physical therapy, you name it. We even did exercises for his hand and arms after the professional therapy was completed to help him return to work faster.

When he finally returned to work, I was concerned when I started to get complaints about his production and work quality. One day I was told he was not working safely or even wearing his PPE. I drove to the job site to find him on the last step of his ladder, wearing no hardhat or glasses. Upon arriving at his job site, I greeted him and sent him home. I told him to be at the office tomorrow at 7 a.m. The next morning, I terminated his employment. He was a hazard to himself and his coworkers. I think he understood.

Looking back on it, I wished I would have been able to make him wait for the other worker to hold his ladder or not use the top steps. I learned that my Safety Program is only as good as what happens when are workers are working unsupervised. I learned that behaviors and not lack of training cause most accidents. And most importantly, I learned that in some cases, you have to let a worker go if they refuse to work safely.

Recently I saw the foreman that I fired on one of our job sites working for a competitor, and we were friendly. I saw him working on his ladder safely.

Takeaway 1: Learn from your mistakes.

When you are just starting out and in charge of a safety program, you may feel like you are constantly under fire. Hence the phrase, "Trial by Fire." You have to assess your professional weaknesses just as much as the deficiencies of your safety program. You have to learn the people in your chain of command, what they expect from you, how they normally react in crises, how they carry themselves, and how and when they like to receive bad news. Anyone can step up and claim success. It is when things don't turn out well that it is time to lead. Leadership in safety requires you to constantly conduct risk assessments and risk management, both for your workers and yourself. Understand cause and effect, anticipate the challenges, plan for the next issue or incident.

As you build trust within your organization, your credibility depends on how you are perceived in both the office and the field. When I had to go to the hospital, I learned about taking ownership of mistakes. I was certainly not capable of preventing the most serious accident that our company has ever had; after all, I was a new safety professional. However, someone on our team was injured, and we needed to understand why this happened.

The world is full of blame shifters, spin doctors, and finger pointers, but there is no place for deceptive, self-preservation tactics in construction safety. When an injury accident happens, ideally, the safety professional needs to approach the challenge objectively. Safety issues are team issues. Take responsibility for making the team better. We want to lead them through the current situation well and set the tone for handling the next one. Everyone on the team, office, and field, needs to know that the safety professional is a reliable and capable resource and is always ready to take the lead to help the team. No one expects you to be perfect because you will not be perfect. But you can and will get better. Just think of it like this, "I am good today, but I will be a better safety professional tomorrow."

With each experience, we should grow and take our lessons learned into the next safety challenge. No need to worry about when the next safety issue will occur; it will come soon enough and usually at the least opportune, most unexpected time. The next time I have to visit a worker in the hospital, I will be focusing on my worker and his family, and I will look to see how we could have prevented the accident and ensure that future incidents are less likely to occur.

Takeaway 2: Never over promise and underdeliver.

Many times we want to promise the big boss something outrageous, he tells us, "We need Zero Accidents,"

"Lower our EMR," or "We need to see results from all of this training." The fact is that we need to be in this for the long haul. New employees will always be a higher risk of injury accidents. Incidents occur more frequently on Fridays or late in the day. In my experience, the veteran, 45-years-old and up foreman, is also prone to complacency and can get injured due to just thinking, "It will never happen to me."

Safety professionals claiming to have a strong safety program comes with inherent risk. How do you take credit for the good years and the good behaviors without accepting responsibility for bad years? Positive trailing indicators are always an easy out in the eternal struggle for the safety professional to prove value. Leading indicators are soft in comparison and always seems to be the go-to option when trailing indicator are not favorable. While we should promise and deliver innovative, engaging training responsive to observed field deficiencies, promising pie in the sky safety goals should be avoided.

When I wanted to reduce back injuries, I introduced ergonomics and lift training. When I saw safety glass violations, I tried to incentivize compliance. Using Safety Incentive gift cards when I see exemplary safety behavior is another method to promote job site safety. But promising that workers will be safer tomorrow than today is not realistic. How do I incorporate the risk factor of hiring 25 new employees in the past two weeks? My promise to the team. "We are trying to get better, help the new workers get up to speed, and join our safety culture."

Takeaway 3: You are your own worst critic.

To be successful in construction safety, the realization that risk is constant and attempts at risk mitigation endless can appear insurmountable. You see your role as one like putting your finger in a hole in the damn as the surging water is on the verge of breaching containment. There are days when you have to shake your head.

Dealing with COVID case clusters on our job sites was one recent example of this. I was convinced that we were on point with our COVID-19 protocol. We had provided options for face coverings, increased site visits, posted signage, and even sent letters to workers' families to reduce COVID cases amongst our employees. Our cases increased. Every worker who complained of the mildest symptom we sent for testing. Still, our COVID cases increased. I wondered why the majority of our cases seemed to be concentrated with one particular Superintendent and even on one particular job.

Some things are just not easily explained.

Many worker behaviors fall into this category. For example, my hospitalized worker. How could a 30-hour trained foreman violate several of the most fundamental ladder safety rules? Was the training deficient? Even more concerning, was the trainer deficient? While it is easy to accept either side, the worker just made bad decisions, or the ladder training could be improved, the best position to take may be to take the middle ground. Workers behave unsafely for many reasons, and safety professionals cannot control all of them. Training is always enhanced by the success or failure stories we share from personal experiences.

A year or so after the hospital incident, I found myself teaching an OSHA-30 Hour class to some concrete workers. The first topic for that Saturday morning class was ladder safety. One student from the previous class was missing. Later in the day, I learned that he placed his ladder on wet plastic, stood on the top rung, and fell and broke his arm. The next week, in his cast, he came back to class and told his story. I thought if I had trained him on ladder safety, he would not have been injured. I could have prevented this accident. Would have, could have, should have.

Takeaway 16: Learn from your mistakes.

Takeaway 17: Never over promise and underdeliver.

Takeaway 18: Be your own worst critic.

Chapter 7

Symbiosis Only Occurs With Great Leadership

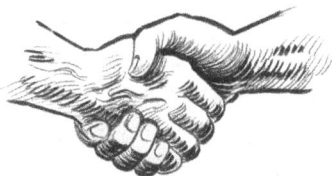

"Buy all the dust masks and respirators that you can!" The company owner proclaimed when he came in the door; all fired up on a Monday morning in late February 2020.

I stood, looking at him, waiting to determine how I would respond. Sometimes he comes up with ideas over the weekend and just "lets them fly" when he sees me first thing on Monday morning. "I saw a program on TV last night. We have to buy as many dust masks and respirators as we can."

I slowly strolled back into my office to create my action plan.

(Note: As a commercial painting company, we routinely use and maintain a closet full of N95 dust masks and half-face respirators with filters for sanding and spray painting. We purchase these through our vendor and restock them monthly. At any given time, we have around 500 units of the two, dust masks and respirators.}

When I shouted over to his office, we already have about 500. He replied, "Double it."

That day I called all of our usual vendors. I was able to buy about 600 more N95 dust masks, and not all of them were the 3M models we were accustomed to buying. At each location, I was told. "That's all I got left." "I only have these two cases." "I only have 100, is that enough?" Three months later, our usual mask vendor is still unable to provide its customers with dust masks or respirators.

It turns out my boss was right again. The next day, 3M, the primary respirator manufacturer, announced a delay in respirator and dust mask orders. Everyone started calling to find dust masks, which became impossible, or they were being sold on the Internet for ten times their normal price.

As the pandemic unfolded, we always seemed to be ahead of the game. My boss and I would talk daily about what I saw on the jobs, what he was hearing, and we would try to anticipate and solve any potential or real problems in the field. The increased attention and interest I received made me feel that my role as Safety Director was more important to the company than ever before.

When we could not find bleach or hand sanitizer, a friend had found a contact to acquire 100 gallons of homemade hand sanitizer, and I ended up using the same contact. The friend drove to my house with his pickup loaded with gallons jugs of homemade hand sanitizer. The next day, I went to the Dollar Store to buy

50 spray bottles to transfer hand sanitizer and distribute them to our job sites.

When the CDC first announced that face covers were recommended, one of my superintendent's wife's sister had started making them. When I told my boss, he said. "Get as many as you can." I drove to her house on a Sunday afternoon and bought 200 face masks she had made at her house. Early on in this crisis, we were handing out facemasks to every employee.

When it seemed like finding any of this COVID-19 PPE was impossible, my boss forwarded a contact through our local Associated Builders and Contractors trade association, and they said they had found a vendor who distributed facemasks, surgical masks, face shields, and hand sanitizer from China. Soon other vendors from other trade relationships, never before involved in the respirator business, were reaching out to us offering the same products with delivery within three or four weeks. I ordered from several of them just to be sure. I wanted to offer multiple options to all of our employees since everyone was not enjoying the facemask policy on job sites and even wearing them when going out in public. Some of the orders took longer than they promised to deliver, but eventually, all of my orders arrived.

Thanks to the vision of my passionate boss and his ability to anticipate our needs, we were well prepared for the pandemic. I was able to support our field supervisors with everything they needed to protect our employees.

Takeaway 1: Great leaders need passion, vision, and problem solving.

"If a leader doesn't convey passion and intensity then there will be no passion and intensity within the organiza-tion."- Colin Powell, 4-Star-General of the U.S. Army

One might wonder why we chose the title, *Symbiotic Safety*. **Symbiosis** can be defined in biological terms as the interaction between two different organisms living in close physical association, typically to the advantage of both, or a mutually beneficial relationship between different people or groups. **Symbiosis** comes from two Greek words that mean "with" and "living." It describes a close relationship between two organisms from different species. In the context of this book, Symbiosis can be considered as the relationships between Safety and Operations, Safety and Field Supervisors, Safety and Employees, and to *the advantage of both*, or a *mutually beneficial relationship between different people* certainly applies.

The leadership of my owner in this situation set the tone for our response to COVID-19. He instituted a Work from Home Policy when he had always resisted this idea when approached about this in the past. I am sure that this was generated by him imagining what would happen if our key personnel were out of commission with COVID-19. This was just another example of how safety can work with the other entities within our company. I felt pressured to set the behavior standard for COVID virus protection. We can't have our safety guy get COVID-19, I would tell myself.

Our Project Managers are still constantly bombarded with requests for our COVID-19 Protocol, Safety Risk Mitigation Plan, etc. We were involved several times a week, redrafting our COVID-19 policy to accommodate the requirements of the City, County, State, GCs, and clients. To the mutual advantage of everyone involved, the relationship at my company between safety, the owner, Project Managers, and Superintendents has been strengthened by our leaders working together and following the vision set by our owner.

Takeaway 2: In times of crisis, no job is more important than taking care of your team.

Effective *leaders* understand their team's circumstances and distractions, but they find ways to engage and motivate, clearly, and thoroughly communicating important issues. Our reaction to COVID-19 was an example of this team-first approach to problem-solving, but there have been others.

When we confronted a series of back injuries among our foremen, we knew that we could not afford to lose any of these key field managers. They were stubborn and impatient veteran workers. Waiting for the younger workers to carry heavier equipment was not something they were accustomed to. When we communicated to these leaders their value to the team and how the team was impacted if they were out due to back injury, the frequency of lift training classes went up, and the injuries went down.

Stilt safety was another example of a team-first strategy. We used to have workers fall off stilts and suffer sprains and strains due to falls incurred while taping and floating. The problem seemed to be increasing. I treated too many injuries with ice and Ibuprofen and felt like I was not being heard about the importance of the hazards of working on stilts. The workers seemed to avoid cleaning their work area before they started work and especially during their workday. They would allow mud to fall on the floor, continue working if other trades left debris in our work area, or take unnecessary risks while walking on stilts. When one day, a well-known subcontractor fell from his stilts and broke his leg, our stilt users paid attention. I explained how he was out for 12 weeks, with a record of no injuries for more than 25 years, and a single screw on the floor made him fall and break his leg. For several years now, we have not had any reported stilts-related injuries. We reinforced our stilt safety policy and trained our workers annually.

Clear, early, and constant communication from leadership will not only address current issues, but it also sets a precedent and level of trust for the future. When leaders react and communicate quickly regarding identified problems, your team can come together and effectively address the issues.

Takeaway 3: Great leadership emerges when problems are identified.

To live through troubled times and emerge stronger, you must create belief in the new vision, align actions, bring people together, and turn fear into excitement. Throughout the years, we have grown from new leaders to good leaders. During challenging times, some people will show great leadership. This is the result of learning from positive and negative experiences. Certainly, the most challenging times can be the most formative, but sometimes when there is no crisis, we become complacent and even begin to doubt the abilities of our leaders.

What is important to avoid when difficult problems arise? Sometimes we tend to criticize, blame, make assumptions, even withhold information or express softball criticism. Tackle the hard stuff first, directly and without hesitation. If they don't know they are creating a problem, they won't know they have to fix it. You can follow up with encouragement and praise to soften the blow without confusing the message.

For example, I have observed the quality of our Tool Box Safety Classes has suffered in the past six months. This may be due to having no injuries over the past few years, or maybe it's the COVID-19 pandemic. Each foreman has to act as a leader and take ownership of our job sites. I know that their focus is to progress toward job completion and deal with manpower issues, but safety has to be on their plate as well. Rather than be critical of my superintendents for not turning in weekly sign-in sheets, I have decided to observe each foreman conducting their weekly Tool Box Safety Class. I want the superintendent to observe, as well. I contribute to the presentation and ensure they are asking the comprehension questions to the topic, and having workers answer them, not just read the answers that I have provided. This way, when I do identify quality issues with our training, I critique the foreman and say I will come back in the next few weeks to see your improvements.

It is important to evaluate each employee on their own strengths and weaknesses, using a clear standard that is fair and equal for all. Base your comparisons on an ideal, not any one person, as your standard. Instead of "Why can't you give your classes like Jose?" Take the time to work with each team member to perform at their personal best. While this is time-consuming, showing the person they are a priority will motivate them to deliver more effective training and elevate their status and improve their leadership.

Takeaway 19: Great leaders needs passion, vision, and problem solving.

Takeaway 20: In times of crisis, no job is more important than taking care of your team.

Takeaway 21: Great leadership emerges when problems are identified.

Chapter 8

Why is Communication so Difficult? (Barriers to Communication)

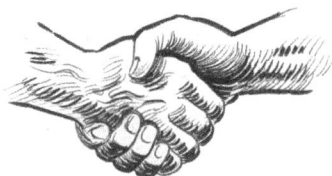

I walked down the dimly lit hallway of the new school, and the first five of my painters I saw were not wearing safety glasses. Say it isn't so. Not again. I thought as I started writing down names. Miguel, David, Jose, Gerardo, and Francisco. Why can't these guys understand that they have to wear safety glasses? We tell them every day. It is not a language barrier. Am I missing something?

I had purchased lunch for our crew on the previous Friday, intending to thank them for their work. After lunch, I made the declaration to them as they captively sat in the shade, avoiding the sweltering Texas heat, that we were not up to standard on this job site with respect to wearing safety glasses. I gently but firmly stated any safety violation by our employees would result in being sent home for the day. In my estimation, my foreman and superintendent had allowed the situation to become out of control. Some claimed that the heat, dirty glasses, the COVID-19 face-covering steaming them up, and the fact that the GC did not seem to mind all made not wearing safety glasses necessary and even acceptable.

I saw this as a challenge to our safety program. The credibility of my foreman and our management team's integrity was at stake. The other 13 workers in other areas of the job site were wearing their safety glasses, why not these guys in the hallway? We had to take a stand, draw a line in the sheetrock dust, make an example of somebody that would surely communicate the message that we were serious and they were not going to get away with this. This was a conspiracy.

But was it really a conspiracy? I know that my workers have a difficult job and an even more challenging home life. Their families at home and those in Mexico or Honduras all have many needs that my workers, who are the alpha breadwinners for their extended families. Many workers put in a 50-60 hour workweek. It is hot, dirty work, and the idea of intentionally trying to undermine our safety program is unrealistic. We just need to communicate better and encourage our workers when they do a job, more coaching less policing. However, there are times when blatant disregard for safety must bring appropriate consequences.

I walked out of the building with my foreman, and I could see his head was down, and he felt discouraged. I said we could not continue to have me tell everyone that they have to wear their safety glasses if you are not going to enforce the rules when I leave. He lifted up his safety glasses and said, "Yo se, Yo se. Es mi culpa. Solo es que necesitamos primear los pasillos hoy y no puedo mandar estos cinco a casa porque solo los únicos que están primeando." (I know. I know. It's my fault, I just can't send these five home today because I need to finish priming these hallways today and these five are the only ones priming.)

I told him that at least one person is going home today. I think it should be Francisco. He has had other safety issues lately, and it would make a good example for the others to send him home. My foreman said I can't just send one of the five home. Everyone will think it is personal and an attack on him. We should send all five home.

This surprised me. I asked, "But what about finishing your priming today?"

"We can finish it tomorrow," he replied.

I then called our Superintendent to update him on the situation and tell him our plan. He said, "That's good. I just need you personally to do it, not the foreman."

I said no, this is for our foreman to do. It is his responsibility. If I do it, our workers will think that I am the only person enforcing the rules. "Ok," the Superintendent said, "you stay and be a witness. We always need a witness."

I said, "No, our foreman needs to do it alone."

My Superintendent replied, "Ok, I will come out and talk to everyone at lunch."

Again, my foreman said no that he wanted to do this alone. My foreman then made an even more surprising statement, "I studied Human Resources in Mexico. I agree. I need to send them home by myself. If I explain to everyone why I am doing it, it will go better."

Finally, my Superintendent also agreed or at least supported the decision. We wanted to make it easier for him, not more difficult. I left him there, and at lunch that day, about an hour later, he sent the five workers home. They all returned the next day wearing their safety glasses.

Takeaway 1: Situational bias based on past experiences.

It feels like I fight the battle of making workers wear safety glasses every day. I make them readily available each time I walk a job site. I carry several extra pairs with me. I even allow my workers to select the color and style of safety glasses they prefer (and provide several different and reasonably-priced alternatives). I usually encourage and gently nudge them when I find them not wearing safety glasses. But why is this such a constant problem? Am I missing something? They are simply trying to complete their work as assigned by my foreman. I get that, but can't safety just become part of their daily routine.

Once a worker asked me how many of your employees have ever lost an eye? Gone blind? I replied, "Zero."

How many have ever suffered a severe eye injury? I replied, "Zero." I added, "I have had two in 15 years that had to use the eyewash from their first aid kit."

Not exactly smoking gun level evidence to compel a behavior change.

Many workers have had inconsistent experiences with safety and especially wearing safety glasses. Some companies don't require them or even issue them. General Contractors may be on one extreme or the other; some will write you up for a safety violation if you do not wear them. Others don't even require the GC's own employees to wear them. Still, others will send you home for the day the first time you do not wear your safety glasses even if you just take them off to clean them! This seems to be like speed limit enforcement. Everyone will admit they speed, but rarely if ever, receive a ticket for doing so. Then after they receive a ticket, they drive more slowly for a while.

One day I was driving through Temple on I-35 with a pack of about ten other cars. Yes, we were speeding. Probably going about 80 mph in a 65 mph zone. Suddenly, the speed limit changed to 55. We kept going together in a pack at about 80 mph. When I first saw the motorcycle cop on the shoulder, I thought we might have road herd immunity, but as soon as we passed him, his lights turned on. I was in the front, middle section of the pack. He began to pass the cars from the group, as one by one each pulled over and awaited their ticket. But the motorcycle cop kept going. Finally, I was the last car, and he pulled up to me, motioning that I move to the side of the road. Incredulously, I pulled over. He slowly sauntered up to me wearing his Frank Poncherello polarized cop shades,

"Good afternoon, Sir. Is there a problem?" I asked.

"You in a hurry? He asked.

"No, Sir."

"I need to see your driver's license, insurance, and registration."

I quickly found them and handed them to the law enforcement officer. In my mind, I kept asking myself, Why me? Why me? How do you pick me instead of the ten other cars driving the same speed?

I had to ask him. "Sir, how did you just pick me out of the group of cars?"

He stopped writing my ticket in his little metal-ticket book and looked down over his cool-cop shades. He asked, "You ever gone dove hunting?

"Yes," I said.

"You shoot all of the doves?"

"No." I could see where this story was going.

"You usually just get one when you shoot?"

"Yes," I mumbled.

"Well, you're my dove."

When a standard is set and implemented with unclear communication and conflicting, sporadic, or non-existent enforcement, it is doomed to fail. Are there no consequences, some consequences, or always consequences for violating a rule? Many workers are accustomed to being told to follow rules of all kinds that are not actually followed. For example, Don't bring food and eat on the job site. Don't leave your water bottles lying around. Don't smoke on the job site. Don't use the top two steps of the ladder. Don't park over here, park over there. Wear your hard hat. Wear your harness. Wear your safety glasses. Our decisions to behave according to the safety rules or not, many times, depend on what has happened to us or others around us when they do not follow the rules. If workers are conditioned to comply with rules because they are part of a safety culture, they will. But if their experiences have proven it's ok not to follow the rules, a challenging barrier to safety communication exists and will have to be removed through establishing a new standard of behaviors. Trust is essential for true dialogue, and without it, free flow of information and the best possible decisions are nearly impossible.

Takeaway 2: What's in it for me?

Originally stated by Henry Ford as a key concept in advertising, we have heard about self-interest driving behaviors for many years. It is used in advertising slogans like, "The Choice is Yours," "Have it Your Way? "Just Do It! We have to confront this mentality daily and answer the question, "What's in it for me?" to create engagement in our safety culture and move past compliance. But are we selling safety? To a certain degree, yes. We certainly need worker buy-in, so we had better offer something that has value for the workers.

With my workers, I have found referencing family has been effective in tying self-interest to safe behavior. Whether that means keeping their job to support their family financially by following the rules or not becoming injured so they can keep working, the issue of family is universal. As workers age and spend more time with a company, many care more about their younger co-workers and that they work for a good, stable company. The point is again clear and should be transparent in our communication about safety; we care about our workers we care about their families. We show this by asking them by name about their family members and trying to keep everyone safe.

I also try to provide individual Safety Awards as an incentive. I use gift cards to catch someone in an exceptionally safe act or when they receive a compliment from a GC or client. It is just intended to let them know that someone is watching and that they see the good things too. Some might argue that this is unnecessary because "They are supposed to be safe and do a good job." Everyone likes recognition of a job well done, and compliments in this world are few and far between. If workers feel appreciated, they are happier and a more productive, safer employee.

Often, compliance-based safety seems impersonal. It is absolute, yes or no, black or white words on a page. By nature, it cannot be personal or subject to individual interpretation or worker issues that justify unsafe behavior due to self-interest. Being in a hurry, not ever having been injured before, cutting corners, a myriad of distractions starting with cell phones, all of these and more could be used to defend unsafe behaviors, and all are behavioral causes of accidents. As safety professionals, we have to keep our focus on the big picture, our safety culture. This provides us a guiding imperative to build trust through relationships, communicate well, and answer the most common question, why? The Who, What, Where, and When answers are usually self-explanatory. While the "How" Is the toughest question to answer, this is left for the safety professional to ponder and plan with all available resources at his disposal and discuss at safety conferences and safety meetings. Why do we do what we do? We do it for you to keep you safe.

Why did my foreman send five people home? Not to punish them, but to keep them safe. In the future, he will have to show them he cares about them in other ways besides just punishing them for unsafe behaviors.

Takeaway 3: Assumptions lead both parties away from clear communication.

What does the typical construction worker think when someone recognizes him performing an unsafe behavior? I thought you just like to get people in trouble, you just want to prove you are doing your job, you just don't like people, you feel more important telling people what to do, you're part of management, not part of us.

What does the typical construction safety professional think when he sees a worker performing an unsafe behavior? Not again, more low hanging fruit, are these guys ever going to learn? Is this a test? Is someone taking a video of me to see how I will react to this? Do they do this intentionally just to piss me off? Now I know why this guy is in construction?

We all have assumptions about behaviors that come from previous experiences that lead us to erroneous conclusions. We often create our own story and fill in all the missing parts from previous bad experiences we have had or hear about from others. How could this possibly lead to better communication? It does not. What it does is create a bias, yet another barrier to communication. The trick is to let the facts create the story. If there are missing parts, seek out more facts through communication and try not to use any assumptions. Granted, this is easier said than done.

I assumed my foreman would want to make an example of the worker who had a recent history of other safety violations. I assumed that he would want me to send the workers home. My superintendent assumed that I should be present or that he should explain to our workers why we did what we did. These are assumptions that lead to unsuccessful action plans and poor results.

We also attempt to speculate about motive, which is a slippery slope. Unless someone tells you directly, your guess about why they did what they did is simply a guess. Successful guessing does not create a productive strategy. Both parties need to reach common ground, for example, keeping everyone safe, completing the project on schedule, making a profit, 100% fall protection, etc. When this goal is shared, and the focus can be established on a mutually desirable objective, communication will generate better results. I ask you to step back and look at your perspective and the worker's perspective. If a third party would think both sides are being reasonable and trying to accomplish an agreed-upon objective, you may be communicating clearly.

Takeaway 22: Situational bias based on past experiences.

Takeaway 23: What's in it for me?

Takeaway 24: Assumption lead both parties away from clear communication.

Chapter 9

Creating an Opportunity for Communication to Thrive

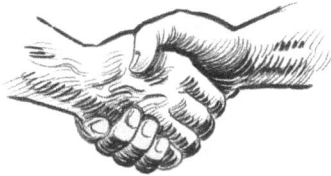

In early March, before COVID-19 changed the world, the Safety Director for a large general contractor asked me for a Job Site Protocol for COVID-19. He said we now require all subcontractors to provide this by Monday. Additionally, you need to appoint a COVID-19 Safety Monitor (CSM) on the job site to enforce the protocol. Shortly after that, the Project Manager for the job asked our Project Manager for the protocol, and the Superintendent for the project asking our Superintendent for the same. I thought that the GC might have been out in front of COVID-19 because they are based in Atlanta, home of the CDC.

I reached out to some of my fellow Safety Directors at GCs and Safety Consultant types regarding what this COVID-19 Protocol was, and no one had confronted this yet. The next day I heard that from a friend that the State of Texas jobs required a COVID-19 protocol as well. He forwarded me his version that included a list of CDC protocols and a health survey sign-in form that each person on the job site had to sign daily. After I created a modified bilingual version of this, I sent it to the GC Safety Director and forwarded copies to several colleagues so they could be prepared for the flurry of imminent requests. A few weeks later, the world changed.

By late April, every General Contractor had corporate, state, county, and city versions of COVID-19 protocols, and somehow all of the job sites remained open in Central Texas. A couple of jobs shut down for a week or so, but with the exception of travelers and nursing homes, Central Texas seemed to be "flattening the curve." After a few weeks, I acquired hand sanitizer, five versions of face masks, disinfectant, and doled these out at each of our jobs and to our superintendents like a COIVD-19 Safety Santa Claus. Communication was exceptionally efficient within our company during this crisis, even though we had a diverse age group of workers ranging in age from 18 to 55. Our office employees had converted in mid-April to 90% working from home with surprising ease. The absence of face to face communication seemed to increase the efficiency of our calls, texts, and emails.

It was the Saturday morning of Memorial Day Weekend, and it started with a conference call with one of my superintendents and project managers about a positive COVID-19 case. The project manager and superintendent said, "We have a worker who tested positive for COVID, what should we do?"

The fact that our first case was also the first case on this large project with two GCs seems ironic. I was about to contact both GCs for the project and was certain of only one thing: the affected worker would not be returning to work on Tuesday. After that, I was hopeful that I could receive clear guidance on what to do with my other workers on the site. Who needed to know about this? What were the conditions of my workers returning to work? I was also concerned about HIPPA rules. How could we protect the rights of this worker when he eventually returned to work? Was his doctor going to provide us documentation of his positive test? Why didn't my worker complain of the three most common symptoms of COVID; cough, fever, and difficulty breathing?

Over the next few hours, I exchanged twenty phone calls, five texts, and three emails on this issue. The first GC did not respond to a call or email but did respond within 10 minutes to my text. The second GC did not respond to my call but did call after I texted. According to my workers, the clinic that called my worker on Saturday morning did not answer my call, and I emailed and left a phone message. My 45-year-old worker answered my call each time immediately. Then I started my series of updates to our company's owner.

The initial facts that I had available On Saturday were as follows:

The worker was asymptomatic on the job for two days (Monday and Tuesday) and had no fever, no cough, no difficulty breathing, or other symptoms at the start of each day.

The worker did not come to work on Wednesday due to feeling body aches and headaches.

The worker felt more aches on Thursday and was tested for Covid-19.

The clinic called the worker on Saturday morning and reported a positive COVID test and said they would email him the documentation for the test on Monday (Memorial Day).

The worker painted doors and frames on five floors of a 33 story building alone; he was not within 6 feet of anyone for more than 15 minutes on both days

I kept my boss updated hourly as the GC Safety Director sought corporate guidance from his office in Atlanta. Ultimately, it was determined that the worker should be quarantined for 14 days, have a negative COVID TEST, and be asymptomatic and could then return to work on June 8, if these conditions were met. We would pay this worker to stay at home. The other six workers who had been on the job site could return to work on Tuesday and be tested for fever as required by the new protocol. Sunday, the floors where our employee worked were to be deep cleaned by the GC's cleaning service.

I texted the first GC to complete the communication loop and called the project manager and owner with the final decision. He seemed genuinely thankful for being responsive and closing the communication loop with all parties. I texted the superintendent, who initiated the call and called the worker one last time to request documentation of his test result on Monday when he received it. For some reason, I felt like the communication on this event was exceptional. Everyone was responsive and reasonable. Was it because we are all at home and could concentrate on this challenge? Was it the gravity and novelty that having our first COVID case brought? Was it the lack of 50 other whirling peas of issues during a normal workday? I could not say definitively. It just seemed pleasantly surprised that on a Saturday morning, on a holiday weekend, seven people could communicate and work together well when they needed to do so.

Takeaway 1: Today's construction safety professional can no longer be a compliance ambassador for OSHA.

As construction safety professionals, we normally spend our time answering questions like: What does OSHA say about this or that? Is what we are doing safe? What is our EMR? Can the GC make us do that? Can you complete these safety documents?

We are now thrust into the limelight, with the new COVID era, the safety professional needs to step up. Yes, OSHA still has important things to say, but the world and the role of construction safety professionals have permanently changed. We are no longer just the guardians of compliance with OSHA's CFR 1926 Construction Safety Standard. We cannot ignore that the normal isn't normal anymore. In fact, the new normal is still unknown. Essential and non-essential overnight became part of our new post-COVID lingo, and fortunately, construction is essential. Do people actually believe they have the right not to wear a mask if they don't want to? Do we think that at some arbitrary near future date, all of this will go away? Is social distancing possible in meetings, training, movie theaters, buffets, attending major sports events? Will these all be things Pre-COVID? Will we talk about life moving forward as before COVID and after COVID?

As safety professionals, we cannot just stand by like Walmart greeters waiting for the newest OSHA COVID Standard. The COVID world has moved the Center for Diseases Control to the forefront. To a depressing and even numbing level, for some of us, our daily lives are inundated with COVID data. Worldwide death count, US case count, city case count, county case count, clusters of cases. What famous person has COVID? Which famous person died from it? What drug is the President taking? Is he wearing a mask? For others, they walk around like the first group is crazy. COVID is a conspiracy, Bigfoot, or the boogeyman. But with more than 1,000,000 dead, I am unsure of how anyone can take this position. I think that is called denial.

We have heard that a concerned chorus is asking, "Is the construction industry doing enough to protect all of these exposed workers? As unlikely as it would have been just a few months ago, construction seems to not only have weathered the storm but emerged as one of the strongest industries, other than PPE manufacturing and healthcare in this new COVID era. The moment has arrived for the safety professional. We have to respond to this challenge and show our COVID safety protocols are exemplary, consistently enforced, and a fundamental component of our safety cultures.

The impact of COVID reminds me of the impact of 9/11 on our country. I was teaching at the University of Texas at the time, and someone entered the classroom and said that the World Trade Center was burning due to two jets crashing. I just kept teaching. Law enforcement psychologists have documented that in active shooter scenarios, when an active shooter enters a room, 30 percent of the people in the room do nothing, 40 percent will look around to see what everyone else is doing. The other 30 percent will implement an action plan. Unfortunately, my mind was in the first group (Do Nothing) and remained there until I traveled by plane for the first time after the incident. I vowed to be more aware of the world as I went from rookie to seasoned safety professional.

When I received news about our first employee who tested positive for COVID, I had my chance to shine for our company. Safety professionals have to be in the third group with respect to COVID and give more to our management team and help our employers move forward. We need to explain the science and put the CDC guidelines and county and city protocols in layman's terms. Simplify and gently correct when we drive up to a job site and see guys two feet apart eating lunch. Mentor and advocate and show and tell everyone (including our workers) that we are protecting our workers.

Takeaway 2: Generational differences create a need for different communication strategies Baby Boomers (born 1945-1964), Generations X (born 1965-1976), Y (Milenials-born 1977-1995), and Z (born after 1996.

As I reflected on our first COVID case, I was reminded of the challenges of multi-generational communication. On that Saturday morning, we were problem-solving, informing, training, educating, and updating people who were from four different generations at the same time. We must be inclusive of the preferred communicative styles of employees and use multiple sources to accommodate these diverse styles, especially due to the importance of implementing COVID protocols.

The superintendent who called, is 38 years old. He normally communicates by text and carries two phones. When I call him, he answers, "What's up?" the translation of which is "What's wrong?" Over the past ten years, I have learned that if he calls me, something is wrong, or he needs something from me. When the 30-40 group responds to a group text, it will normally be a gif or emoji with some tongue in cheek message responding to the current issue. The fact that he initiated this call meant that a serious issue was at hand.

For example, as a generalization, the Baby Boomers (55 years old and Up) prefer face to face communication. Generation X (35 to 45 year-olds) prefer e-mails and phone calls. Millennials (Generation Y 25 to 35 year-olds) prefer texting and Generation Z or Snowflakes, the 24 and under group is more visual and prefer images, video with brief texts and is also much more sensitive.

Attention spans and social needs vary as well. But face to face contact trumps all communication. My point here is that we have to acknowledge these differences, learn the preferences of our coworkers, and continue to distribute COVID information and all safety communication through various formats to be most effective. If you provide a paper document with your face mask, hands, and hand sanitizer, could it also be sent out concurrently in an email and text with a link to the CDC guidelines in Spanish and English and a Youtube video on correct hand washing technique, how to wear a mask and social distancing? It is also important to have ongoing dialogue and to build trust. Some GCs, subcontractors, companies, job sites will enforce protocol better than others. If someone observes breaches of protocol, let's think of using these as teachable moments and positively reinforce how we appreciate our employees for working safely.

Increased awareness of communication preferences is a necessity for the safety professional toolbox. You may notice certain types of communication receive less feedback and others more. You may be complimented on some more than others. Analyze the trends and recognize the preferences. This simple practice will make for more successful communication and a more effective safety culture.

Takeaway 3: The COVID-driven new normal is improving safety in commercial construction.

I have observed an encouraging safety trend in the COVID era. For the most part, my job sites seem safer. No science for this conclusion, just an observation. I believe this comes from the fact we have substantial buy-in to follow COVID protocol. We are talking about COVID safety all the time. Safety is safety.

A 10-year electrician who has never fallen off a ladder may be less than enthusiastic about being preached to by his safety professional for not using the top steps of a ladder. But if he knows that people are dying from COVID and he is told wearing a face covering, washing his hands, and keeping social distance protects him from COVD, he willingly complies.

Information about COVID safety is everywhere. This new awareness of this health hazard may have heightened the recognition of all workers that we, as an industry, need to be safe. Not just to protect ourselves, but because people are watching, and for a while, we were one of the few industries that did not stop working. Our mentality that "We want you to work safely and go home safely to your family" has more traction than ever before. I feel like it gives construction workers a sense of pride to know they are still going to work every day, literally out in the trenches, at a time of post-Depression high unemployment and a growing stay-at-home work-force.

In the pre-COVID world, I would attend job fairs and hear high schoolers saying, "My dad said, "If I can't go to college, then I could work in construction. Anyone can do that." Well, not a warm feeling for the industry, but we have many options for career paths in construction, and we have many jobs available. Our ability to promote construction safety and now COVID-safety to these potential recruits will substantially impact our near future. We had a progressively worsening man-power shortage before COVID, and we don't need to make it any worse by having COVID clusters in the construction industry, the reputation for being unsafe, or workers complaining about how their employers are not protecting them.

Workers today seem more aware and more engaged with safety than ever before. I am receiving more questions through texts, calls, emails, and face to face. Some of my workers wanted to know if they are safe, especially after our first COVID positive worker. Performing recent job site inspections has shown me that wearing masks, a very new requirement, is working. We had only one worker test positive, but I rarely have to ask a worker to put on his mask.

It may be helping that I have chosen to offer more options for PPE than ever. If the worker wants a surgical mask, a cloth face covering, a KN95 mask (the Chinese version of the N95 with similar performance for COVID protection), a gaiter, or even wear their own version of a face covering, I am supportive. Weekly, I offered replacements and all of the options. We reserve N95 masks for sanding sheetrock, but slowly our workers have found that the KN95 and cloth masks work just as well for our purposes. More importantly, the KN95 version is available. Everyone likes to be able to make their own decisions. We have successfully employed this same approach, offering options of color and style with safety glasses. If I like my safety glasses, I will wear them more. Therefore, I am safer.

Takeaway 25: Today's construction safety professional can no longer be a compliance ambassador for OSHA.

Takeaway 26: Generational differences create a need for different communication strategies Baby Boomers (born 1945-1964), Generations X (born 1965-1976), Y (Milenials-born 1977-1995), and Z (born after 1996.

Takeaway 27: The new normal will elevate the role of the safety professional in Commercial Construction.

Chapter 10

Mutual Understanding

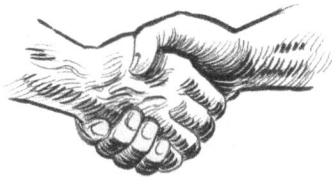

The Safety Warning Near Miss e-mail was awarded to ten people. Seven were from the GC's company, and three from my company (a commercial painting subcontractor), include the President, Project Manager, and Safety Director. In green, in 24 Arial Font, the notice read: "Risk Level: LOW" accompanied by a photo of my employee on stilts standing near a utility cart, next to a fire extinguisher stand with several sets of cable on the floor and visible barricade signs pushed over.

This was part of the quarterly *Safety Bonus* system that this GC had established. Each GC Superintendent had to catch a subcontractor violating a safety rule, take a picture, and fill out a form. If you completed three of these by the end of the quarter, you received your safety bonus. If not, it was deducted from your paycheck. This made the end of the quarter the most common time when these warnings were sent...trying to make the quarterly Safety Bonus deadline.

I had had enough. This was my foreman, trying to tape and float in an area that he barricaded, and the other trades continued to enter his work area, remove his barricade, and create hazards for him. We had already complained that the other trades were not following the rules in the past two meetings. They merely said, "Tight schedule. Gotta get it done. No time to wait around."

They were not respecting the barricaded work area rule that had been repeatedly stressed in the pre-con meeting. I was not happy. My project manager shouted across the hall, "Did you see that email?" The president added, "You need to handle this," which is always nice to know that we were guilty before proven innocent. "It's always the painter's fault," my president added for good measure.

I was determined to put an end to this unfounded harassment and set this assistant superintendent straight. I planned to go to the job site the next morning and talk to him and get this hammered out. We needed his support following their rules.

The next morning I was in the office, and an e-mail arrived. I opened it and saw it again, "Safety Warning Near Miss, Risk Level: LOW." This time it was the GC's superintendent, an unusually calm and reasonable superintendent compared to most of his peers. His email to our project manager included the following:

"This behavior cannot continue. I will not stand for another safety violation of your workers on stilts. You need to come down here and give them a Stilt Safety class. If I catch them breaking the rules again, they will not be allowed to use stilts on this job."

That settles it, I thought. I grabbed my Dura Stilts Safety Class brochure and Sign-In Sheet, and off I went to settle the score. On the way, I thought there must be something else to this. We have worked with stilts for years and never received a complaint from this GC. As it turns out, I was correct. I decided to tune down my fight or flight reflex and collect intel at the job site.

Upon arrival, I asked the GC's Superintendent if I could use their conference room. I gathered my team of six employees, all of whom were complaining about how unfair it was that they were in trouble about the stilt safety rules. It seemed to me this was more an administrative issue, an enforcement issue rather than one of improper use of equipment or a safety issue. But we proceeded to review the Dura Stilt Safety Rules and Do's and Don'ts. I told my team to keep up the good work, and promised to help make this problem go away. I then went up to the third floor to see the superintendent and present him with my training materials and sign-in sheet.

As I stepped off the elevator and looked down the hall, there sat a tired looking superintendent seated in front of a white plastic folding table on a metal chair. (Make no mistake, there are few jobs more difficult than being a superintendent on a commercial construction job site.) As I approached, he looked up to greet me and receive the documents from my class. He thanked me and said my guys always do a good job. I was confused.

Then it happened. "Your guys are really not the problem. We have had 12 accidents on stilts this year from other painting companies. We are just getting tired of painters ignoring the rules." I thought of many things I wanted to say at that moment, but now was not the time for most of them.

"I understand," I said. Could you just help enforce the barricade rules for my guys on stilts? If they try and are ignored by the other trades, could you help them enforce the rules?"

"Sure, he replied. Thanks for coming out. We like working with you guys."

A few days later, I received another email sent to the group of 10 with a photo. "Here is your worker working safely on stilts. Good job! Thanks for being safe!"

It was the first time in 10 years we had received a compliment from this GC.

Takeaway 1: Upon receiving information regarding a "Safety Violation," construction safety professionals should always seek out the facts and the circumstances before rushing to judgment and developing an action plan.

As a safety director for a subcontractor, I am always challenged when I initially react to a reported safety violation against one of my employees. The us vs. them mentality sets in. On the one hand, I know that general contractors have to report job site behaviors that are not compliant with CFR 1926, OSHA's Construction Safety Standard. But on the other hand, I know the training my workers have received, and I'm confident that my foreman ensures that our workers work safely 99 percent of the time. When I hear that we have violated job site safety rules, in an area that we have consistently trained, I am both skeptical and hopeful and think, "Who did it this time?" or "What are we getting blamed for this time?" (Depending upon whether I am feeling cynical or optimistic on a given day.) But initial reports are often filled with partial truths or missing critical information and only present one perspective.

I know that my workers are knowledgeable regarding the rules. I also know that they are stubborn when it comes to the administrative logistics of efficiently managing multiple trades in our work areas when others do not follow job site safety rules. (construction sequencing is not pretty. For some GCs, it is like making sausage. It is not a simple task to juggle demanding clients and dynamic schedules with subcontractors who have limited manpower and windows of opportunity to be on a specific job site.) When confronted with safety challenges, some of our foremen will dig their heels in and "get'er dun" or try to avoid the issue completely. This leads to risk-taking and a potential safety violation or slowing down production and waiting until our superintendents arrive to start playing the blame game. Others will push back and get frustrated with the perceived bias of the GC Superintendent or the other trades not following the GC's safety rules. Safety on job sites sometimes is used as a Sword/Shield strategy; push the strength of your safety record to win the contract and at the beginning of the job and then provide your training documentation when GCs question it and defend yourself with your previous success stories.

The facts of a situation may be that the worker in question was observed violating a safety rule. However, do we consider the worker's intentions? What actions or behaviors occurred prior to the alleged infraction? Did he intend or attempt to comply? Was he forced to choose production over safety by the GC or another trade? Did other GC superintendent personnel look the other way, encourage unsafe practices to complete work on schedule and only issue a safety violation after the safety professional arrived at the job site? The facts also may be conflicting.

In the story with stilts, here are five facts not mentioned in the original email:

My worker worked in an area with obstructions in his work area after he started working and had barricaded his work area. This violated the GCs Stilt Safety Policy. But the Controlled Access Zone was not obstructed when he began working.

The other trades in our work area had removed the barricades that we had established in our CAZ to facilitate their work in the same area due to the "tight schedule."

My foreman had requested support from the GC superintendent to enforce the Stilt Safety Policy after the barricades were removed and did not receive it due to "scheduling issues."

The GCs Stilt Safety Policy had failed multiple times on other job sites, with other painters, resulting in serious injuries that same year.

The written threat to deny our use of stilts on the job site had nothing to do with the unsafe use of stilts by my employees.

Knowing these facts helped me to communicate with the GC superintendent and create a safer job site. He just wanted to avoid future worker injuries and run a safe job site so that his safety personnel would not badger him for being out of compliance. I saw it as an opportunity to give refresher training in Stilt Safety, improve our relationship with this GC for this job site as well as future work and provide a positive example of a problem-solving base on good communication from my employees and advocating their viewpoint while at the same time meeting the needs of the GC superintendent. I think that we often forget that in many ways, we are on the same team. Aren't we both trying to satisfy the client, build on time, and make money? Is it possible and necessary that both parties do so? Communication is best when we do not anticipate motives, but rather seek out more facts to make the best decision possible.

Takeaway 2: Occam's Razor, the simplest explanation for the problem is usually correct, but not always; there are infrequent exceptions.

The safety violation, in this case, was not as it appeared. Its causes were not intentional behavior, lack of training, or expediency. The causes were lack of communication, lack of enforcement of administrative policies, and less than optimal construction sequencing/schedule of trades. While these are common issues in construction, they should be immediately treated when they arise. The idea that is the new normal implies acquiescence with conditions that are more easily corrected at the outset rather than waiting for the inevitable confrontation and test of wills. I know that sometimes my superintendents do not feel that they have the time to confront GC's concerns at the outset. In their mind, they put out other fires first, and safety issues can be put on the back burner. When it reaches a boiling point (injury accident, documented safety violation write-up, or near-miss), they will involve their safety professional.

The conditions in this instance had been going on for more than a week. The back and forth between the other trades and GC was not resolving the problem. From my perspective, the decisions made to remedy this particular situation were driven by a long-term relationship with this GC, multiple current and future projects with this GC, and a knowledge of their safety program and my confidence in my foreman.

Choosing to be proactive rather than reactive once again proved to be a more effective response compared to the customary finger-pointing, and he said/she said exchange. I think that frazzled GC superintendents respond well to genuine efforts to problem solve and focus on a purpose that mutually benefits both parties. But a bait and switch strategy designed solely for the subcontractor's one time need to duck and cover, sabotages future exchanges that could be handled more expediently if they would choose to take the higher road when any potential conflict is identified.

Supporting field personnel is mission-critical and taking the time to meet with my team on-site, face to face, discussing their concerns made them feel satisfied and supported. Then, presenting our perspective and suggestions to the GC superintendent in a calm, fact-based presentation allowed for a better outcome than one that starts with conflict. My 10-year relationship with my foreman, hand-picked by the GC's project manager for this project, urged me to dig deeper before overreacting. Had I refused to provide the Stilt Safety Class or immediately refuted the safety violation, I would have missed the opportunity to create the mutual purpose and trust needed to resolve the issues at hand in the best possible way. The GC's appreciation was evident at the time, as well as in the positive email sent congratulating us on our worker who suddenly was *working safely*.

Takeaway 3: Being correct does NOT mean you will win. Winning is when all parties are

satisfied with the option and that the situation at hand immediately improves.

Safety seems to be black and white; an activity is either performed safely or unsafely. This is what it looks like in a contract or at the office reading an email. When working in the field, situational variables arise, and so do differing opinions. When GC and subcontractor safety professionals work together mutually, agreeable decisions can be made. Time and time again, I find myself sitting in pre-construction safety meetings where project managers are reviewing job site safety requirements that are not consistently enforced in the field. For example, the Controlled Access Zone with barricades for using stilts was addressed multiple times in the pre-con meeting. The GC's project manager, assistant project manager, superintendent, and assistant superintendent separately emphasized Stilt Safety in their presentations. The situation in the field was a disregard for the policy due to production schedule constraints and delivery logistics as two GC were working on two separate projects on a logistically challenged, downtown Austin job site.

Most people are wired to attack or fight back when they perceive an attack when issues arise that were previously considered addressed and therefore resolved. But this is often counterproductive. Many GC Superintendents have to fight all day long, even within their own company at times. They expect to have confrontations with subcontractors and seek to impose their will at all costs. Therefore, safety professionals of subcontractors who seek the "ah-hah" moment where you can blame someone else for a safety issue would be well-advised to work on fixing the problem with a no-fault mentality. Any victory with the battle-hardened GC superintendent will be short-lived, and being adversarial does not benefit the GC/subcontractor relationship for the duration of the job. Their clients give GC superintendents nearly impossible schedules through their project managers, and they cannot explain why the job will not be completed on time when the guys in the office have promised it. Safety requirements customarily take a back seat to production schedule, and budgets and real safety concerns have to be presented when there is a window of opportunity. Offering a lifeboat to the GC superintendent and helping him to appease his safety professionals' concerns sets a tone for more successful outcomes in the next round.

Takeaway 28: Upon receiving information regarding a "Safety Violation," always seek out the facts and the circumstances before rushing to judgment and developing an action plan.

Takeaway 29: Occam's Razor, the simplest explanation for the problem is usually correct, but not always, there are exceptions.

Takeaway 30: Being correct does mean you will win. Winning is when all parties are satisfied with the option, and the situation at hand immediately improves.

Chapter 11

Common Purpose

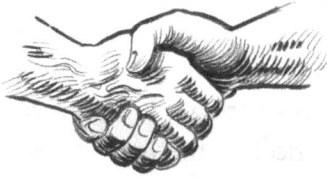

About ten years ago, when we received a contract for a job with a large high tech company in Austin, we had no idea what was in store for us. Rumors had mentioned that we needed a safety budget to work for them, that everyone had to have a background check, badges, steel-toed boots, and that the lunch buffet was exceptional. They also said that they had Ladder Safety Officers, gave away tools to everyone, and had safety equipment and PPE requirements that we had never heard of.

The first day we showed up to start the job, we did not have our badges, so we could not work.

The second day, we had our badges, but we did not have steel-toed boots, so we could not work. The GC said that they had told our PM about this from the time we received the contract, our PM disagreed. I went to buy steel-toed boots for all of our workers, and we missed the orientation. So, we came back on the third day.

The third day the orientation was a 2-hour presentation by several safety professionals from the GC. This was when we learned that all the rumors were true. While there were many new safety policies for us to learn and equipment to buy, our project manager was not a happy camper. To him, this meant less production, more costs, and less profit...but as the safety guy, I was fascinated. This company had taken the concept of a safety culture to a whole new level that I have not seen since. For one example, we actually had to check out a ladder from a ladder safety officer, barricade our work area, have our own ladder competent person at the work area, use a spotter and return the ladder to the ladder safety officer at the end of the day. Everything seemed so positive to the safety guy.

Color-coded JSAs, safety signs, posters, cones all in an unoccupied office building that was being remodeled for a new department. Meetings, trainings, and daily lunches with five separate chefs at cooking stations. Although we could not sit in the same area as the client's employees, construction employees were encouraged to eat lunch in the dining room. After word spread to some of our workers about the boots and lunch, nearly all of them wanted to work there.

Today I would say it all made sense. Their intent was clear: Risk Management and Risk Control as part of a positive safety culture. There was nothing left to chance. All safety compliance requirements were exceeded, all supervision was in place, and behavioral accident causes were mitigated. It was impossible to work on this job site without situational awareness and thinking Safety, Safety, Safety! Safety seemed equal to or more important than the actual construction process. No schedule or production decision was made without considering safety. Every detail of the JSA was followed and inspected by multiple parties. Sometimes safety

feels like a sixth finger, but not on this job. Risk mitigation was a natural result. This safety culture had created
a common purpose. It is one thing to say you care about
your workers, but the effect of showing them you care is
considerably more effective.

They used a Stretch and Flex program in conjunc-
tion with current popular music to start the day. Even
this had fail-safe measures implemented. If you showed
up late, the Stretch and Flex officer would make you do
remedial stretch and flex, and everyone had to take turns
leading the exercises. Sign In sheets were abundant, and
a few of my workers learned this the hard way and were
never late again.

The promised Safety Incentive Lunches were delivered and did not disappoint. At the project mid-
point and upon project completion, a white table cloth,
the chef-served buffet was set up on the same floor as
the work area, and the workers loved it. They loaded
their plates with several different meats, and my workers could return for multiple trips. One of my workers
said to me, "Painters don't eat salads. Good bosses give
workers lunches with lots of meat." Signs all over the
job site said "Thank You for Working Safely," and even
the office folks were invited to come to lunch. Upon
completion of lunch and the dessert buffet table, the
hosts GC and the company thanked the workers for the
efforts and working safely on the project. There was no
mention of how many injuries over how many days because the client was thinking beyond that.

I had attended BBQs in the past, where the number of days without reported injuries was posted on a
banner above the event and mentioned several times
throughout the lunch. "180 Days Accident-Free!" Then
the GC would award 10 to 15 trophies to all of their

team for safety excellence on the project. Not a single thing, other than the lunch was given to the trade workers. The focus here was not just on safety, but it promoted and produced, dare I say it, happy workers. Yes, happy. The ideal positive reinforcement-based safety culture. My employees on other job sites asked to work at this job. At times we risked overmanning the job. Had it not been for the time involved in badging, orientation process, and the steel-toed boot requirement, I would have probably sent many more workers to this job for the experience.

As the second dessert, everyone at the Safety Incentive Lunches received a numbered ticket as they entered the dining area, even the office guys, and this was for the tool drawing. The first time I went, I saw the workers' numbers called. They walked to receive their tool and shake hands with the GC superintendents and safety staff. The tools awarded were power tools, not screwdrivers, and wrenches, and I was sure that only a few of these would be given out. But as time passed, every single person at the lunch received a tool that cost $50 to $200. Like soccer trophies being given out to 3rd-grade soccer players, everyone who showed up got a trophy.

Their message was simple: Be Safe, Work Safe, Go home Safe at the end of the day. When workers understand this, the investment in safety culture seems like it should be the norm for all companies. I always try to recreate this message on our job sites even though without the lunches, boots, and tools, it's more challenging. I think emphasizing the common purpose of worker safety has to be more than just a slogan.

Take Away 1: Changing behaviors, changes attitudes.

This experience reminded me of the important role of a safety culture and how it creates a common purpose. Safety culture has been described as a pattern of behaviors encouraged or punished by a management system over time. When we set out to establish or change a safety culture, we are changing behavior and attitudes. If this experience taught me only one thing, it was that attitude changes follow behavior and this is most effectively accomplished through positive reinforcement. A safety culture consists of many different activities and behaviors. Ladder Controlled Access Zones, Ladder Safety Officers, Stretch and Flex programs, Steel Toed Boot Requirements, JHAs, Safety Incentive Lunches, and more. No matter where you stand in management of the construction food chain (safety professional, Superintendent, HR Manager, Foreman, Project Manager, etc.), you want to change the behavior of the people you work with. The client did not have to tell us they were changing our behavior to change our attitude. The power of their safety culture and positive reinforcement did so seamlessly. The General Contractor on the job had been converted, and they, in turn, converted all of their subcontractors. This indoctrination was a little bumpy at first, but shortly thereafter, we were all part of the the client's safety culture.

From this experience, I learned that we did not have a safety culture at that time. I see the impact of lessons learned from this experience on my safety culture today. We are simply better for it. Every time we confront new safety challenges, I think about this experience. When I review our policies, we continue to try to do things better. All of my foreman and superintendents have 30 Hour OSHA training. All of my new employees have OSHA 10 Hour training. I am an OSHA Outreach Trainer. We now use gift cards to incentivize outstanding safety acts or exceptional leaders. We have foreman meetings, set goals, discuss currents issues with meals, and talk positively about safety achievements. No matter how daunting a pre-con safety contract appears, no job ever meets or exceeds the demands or rewards from the the client's experience.

No doubt, my team pushed back from the first day. Led by our incredulous project manager, who, more than anyone, could not accept that these new safety policies were absolute, undeniable, and part of something bigger than contract documents. The GC on the job had become an agent for a positive safety culture. For example, it took us many failed attempts to master the complexity of their "new to us, color-coded JSA." We would make half-hearted attempts at breaking down our tasks and their associated risks and remediation only to have them returned like a 3rd-grade teacher using red ink on your homework and writing REDO on the top. Other trades would even mentor us and answer our questions. We soon gained a feeling of satisfaction as part of a team when are JSAs were approved, even receiving occasional compliments on them. It mattered to my foreman and superintendent that someone was watching everything we did. Positive reinforcement was responsible for our change in behavior and attitude toward safety.

Takeaway 2: Positive reinforcement works, negative reinforcement is rarely necessary.

Another striking feature of this experience was the lack of yelling, threats of being sent home, or accusations of being out of compliance. No blaming or finger-pointing toward other trades for a tight schedule. No demands for weekend or night work to get caught up. In other words, there was no punishment or negative reinforcement used. All of these acts seem to be a part of most construction jobs, and safety professionals often fall victim to this counterproductive practice. For example, when a GC's safety manager threatens a worker to be sent home or give a written safety violation for not wearing safety glasses, the worker reluctantly puts on his safety glasses, and the safety manager believes he has won. The problem with this approach is when the safety manager leaves, the worker will take off his glasses. Negative reinforcement only produces a short term or immediate behavior change. Why did I not have a single issue with safety glasses on this job site?

This experience focused on safety culture and positive reinforcement. There even seemed to be a positive pressure to be like the other trades. If they could do it, then so could we, I thought. Wearing PPE was just a behavior that you are supposed to demonstrate when you work safely in construction. Failure to wear safety glasses was the singular issue guaranteed to be present on every job we had up until this job. I had observed that the same issue was present with every construction trade. Just as we had changed our behavior and attitude about ladders and JSAs, safety glasses for my employees were just part of how you were supposed to work. Here, safety was not optional. I wanted to apply this concept to all jobs to see if it were truly that simple. Did positive reinforcement generate the desired behavior to be repeated?

Empowered by my recently discovered secret weapon, I found a guinea pig in a new hire. I conducted my normal safety orientation and emphasized PPE as usual, "We wear safety glasses at all times at the job site. I will be conducting job site safety inspections weekly. I expect to see you wearing your safety glasses regardless of what other trades or other employees from our company do."

A few days later, I was on the new employee's job site. When I found him working with five other employees, I was glad to see he was wearing his safety glasses, and unfortunately, my other workers were not. I greeted him and thanked him loudly in front of the group for wearing his safety glasses. Suddenly I pulled out a large Yeti tumbler and presented it to him for working safely. The other workers had stopped to watch the show. Immediately they pulled out their safety glasses from their pockets or around their neck. I started heading back to my truck. One worker approached me, stating, "I am wearing my glasses. Can I get a Yeti tumbler too?"

I said, "Sorry, I only had one today. Maybe next time I show up, you'll be wearing your safety glasses, and I will have another one."

I made it back to the truck, and two other workers had followed me and asked me the same question. I gave the same answer. "I am glad you are wearing your safety glasses. I hope you will be wearing them next time I come to the job site."

For the next few weeks, I found that most of my workers were now wearing their safety glasses, and many asked about the Yeti tumbler. I have had few incidents related to not wearing safety glasses since then and can thank my recent experience for the lesson in positive reinforcement. I try to thank workers for working safely more often than I used to. I am not, however, advocating the blanket use of safety incentives. Current research tells us that workers who are bought off with tangible rewards need continuously increasing incentives, and violations and injuries continue. I advocate using personal rewards like compliments, recognition of positive safety leadership, and genuine appreciation for work done safely. These methods help to ensure that these behaviors and attitudes continue when no one is watching.

Note: This does not discount negative reinforcement in cases where someone deliberately refuses to work safely. A negative safety attitude and non-compliant behaviors sometimes cannot be fixed. Documentation is necessary and progressive discipline requires documentation to establish a path to terminating the employee's position. We cannot allow an employee to put themselves or their co-worker in harm's way due to a lack of regard for safety. But it should be used as a last resort.

Take Away 3: When best practices are an expectation, compliance is never even mentioned.

Over the nine months, we worked at the high-tech company's job site. I never hear the word "compliance" or OSHA Regulations. Worker involvement in safety was expected. The GC asked, "What do your workers think about this?" Their JSA required that the workers help define the steps in the daily tasks and identify the hazards present. There was an actual dialogue about safety each day, and I can honestly say that my team was the highest skilled and least safety-oriented of all of our employees when that job started. I did not know it at the time, but I was learning about the concept of best practices. The lesson was reinforced by Green and Red Scaffold tags, a Competent Person in each area, and Steel-toed boots. Why would we wear steel-toed boots in an office building? Because their policy said so, and at the time, that was good enough for me.

Analyzing job site hazards both before the project started and daily is essential. Also, the paperwork seemed endless. We documented, signed, and submitted more than ever before on that project, and we were asked to correct and clarify regularly. Today I feel like documentation is frequently treated like a checking the box experience. Sometimes we still submit an exact copy of the previous day's JHA even though our scope of work has changed, and no one notices. Several companies have a written job site-specific safety orientation in Spanish that must be read and signed before a worker can enter a job site. The only problem is many of my Spanish speaking workers don't read Spanish well. If I were to ask them about the content of the job site orientation reading, I am sure their retention of the information in that document would be less than 50%. And yet they all sign to have read and understood the safety policies on a given job site.

I think we are often complacent with compliance and settle for it rather than asking the difficult questions. Is it necessary to take these risks? Is there a safer and more economical way to perform this task? Are we sure we are not just doing the same thing in the same way we always have done? Complacency, cutting corners, being in a hurry all are top behavioral causes of accidents and are easily allowed to flourish in the "Just get'er done" world of commercial construction.

I can now appreciate how this high-tech company must have developed its safety culture. They probably learned the hard way that what seems to be good enough, sometimes isn't good enough.

Takeaway 31: Changing behaviors changes attitudes.

Takeaway 32: Positive reinforcement works, negative teinforcement is rarely necessary.

Takeaway 33: When best practices are an expectation, compliance is never even mentioned.

Chapter 12

Maintaining the Course

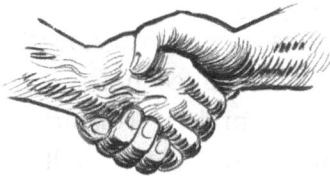

"Anyone can steer the ship. It takes a true leader to chart the course." – John Maxwell

In construction, working for the same organization for over two decades is rare. Upon reflection, there are so many great memories of projects and people. As I look back at some of the first projects with my current employer, my memory is that we have always been very good at what we do. Those projects from 20 years ago were difficult, and our systems and people were prepared for them. All of the early plans we had made for improvement were exactly what the organization needed to enable success in our staff. I am extremely proud of how well we ran those projects 20 years ago.

The other side of those memories is almost funny today. The amount of change in the complexity of projects and the necessary systems in safety are enormous. What was extremely successful 20 years ago would be an abject failure today. Those systems, training, plans, and people were great back then, but without adapting to the circumstances, it would be sad to see today. The only constant is change.

During an interview for a large hospital project, one of the representatives for the hospital asked an important question – "This hospital will not open for four more years. How will your firm help us ensure that when we open, we won't have four-year-old technology in the hospital?" The significance of the question eluded us at first. How is a construction firm able to help you understand emerging hospital technology? Three years later, near the end of the project, we started to understand. The question was really, "How well can you adapt to changes?"

Creating an incredible safety program that achieves all safety goals and creates a symbiotic relationship with all other aspects of the organization is a fantastic achievement. But tomorrow, it is outdated. Planning for the inevitable change is crucial.

Takeaway 1: Adaptability must be built into the safety program.

Intuitively and experientially, you know that change is coming. If you could accurately predict what changes will happen in the next five years, you would quit your job in safety and become a successful stockbroker. We may not know exactly what will change, but we all know that change is inevitable. The successful safety professional is prepared to adapt. Not only prepared for random changes but preplanned. All safety programs should have periodic reviews to assess if the current safety system is the best solution for the current situation. The unsuccessful safety professional will wait until the current system does not work and then react. Schedule periodic reviews of each minor component and the big picture strategies to see if circumstances have changed. Some examples are new technology or tools that could improve safety, integrating safety reports and production reports, or evaluating if anything is too outdated and could be removed. Schedule reviews to evaluate all safety systems.

During the COVID pandemic of 2020, we began to see a sharp increase in the number of people testing positive for COVID-19. We knew our job site protocols were good, and we had numerous spot checks to prove that the guys were complying. Everything that could be done at work was being done and done well. What we could not control was how to get the workers to practice social distancing and wearing face masks while away from work.

Construction safety plans only work when the worker is *AT* work. How could we get all of these guys to continue the safety precautions while off the job? Momma – that's how. We drafted a letter to each worker's family, explaining we needed their help in getting our workers to comply with the COVID safety precautions even away from the job. We mailed the letter, one side in English and the other in Spanish, to each worker's home, addressed to their family. Never in my career have I needed to seek a worker's family to aid in safety functions. But this was the first pandemic I had ever been through. Unusual circumstances will not be solved with the usual solutions. At the risk of jinxing the result, no further COVID-19 cases have been reported in over three months! Not one! That is after 13 cases in June.

How often can we develop a plan, implement it, and it works just like it is supposed to. If there were ever a time to celebrate a success story, this is that time. Moms and wives are highly influential in all families, and this can be especially true in Hispanic families.

Takeaway 2: Maintenance must be built into the safety program.

A large project once had a beautiful illuminated hanging wall feature. It was a statement piece that the architect was extremely proud of. This light feature was going to create a spectacular entrance into the building. The only problem was that there would be no way to ever perform maintenance on the lights inside this hanging wall of glass. The person charged with building maintenance was arguing passionately that the piece had to change. The architect was just as passionate that the piece could not be altered. In the end, the piece was altered so that access could be made inside this hanging glass wall to maintain the light system inside. The architect understood that a perfect design becomes useless if it is not able to be maintained.

Likewise, a safety program starts to deteriorate quickly without maintenance. The most obvious need for maintenance is personnel. When determining how to initiate change within your organization, you must also determine how to maintain that change. The Hawthorne studies 100 years ago proved that workers respond when something new is introduced. They studied how lighting would affect production. What they found was more impactful to sociologists than lighting engineers. When the lighting was increased, production went up. To prove how much this production bump was, they reduced the lighting. Again, production went up. It turns out that workers respond to a new situation, especially if they know metrics are being recorded, much more dramatically than a change in lighting.

This phenomenon means that when you roll out a new safety plan and train everyone, safety will improve. But soon, things become normal, and workers will revert to a "normal mode." There has to be a plan to maintain the program. First, you must train, then you have to have a system to reinforce consistently. Negative reinforcement only works when it's extremely rare. The ongoing safety maintenance must use positive reinforcement along with peer pressure. The new system must become the normal system, or it will fade quickly.

Personnel changes are inevitable. When an entire organization has changed, and every worker has adopted the new safety program as normal, how will the new people learn this? Maintenance of your safety program must include significant consideration of how to incorporate new personnel into the system.

The most difficult part of maintaining a safety program is reminding workers of everything they need to remember. No matter how easily understood and universally received a safety guideline is, if you quit talking about it, it is no longer perceived to be important. When anything is not perceived as important, people will forget about it. Conversely, if you continue to talk about subjects that are universally known and accepted, the messenger gets ignored. The skillful safety professional will understand this and find creative ways to remind workers of safety rules without being a broken record or Captain Obvious.

Takeaway 3: Constant improvement must be built into the safety program.

Success is a subjective word. What is a success for me today would not be something to celebrate 20 years from now. Achieving milestones without an accident or a lowered EMR are easy milestones to track. These trailing indicators are not great indicators of success. Neither are most leading indicators. The number of observations or safety meetings are only indicators of effort, not results. Employee perception surveys could be valuable, but they are easily manipulated. When I was young, I taught full-day safety classes. The classes were on Saturday, and the students expected to be in the classroom until 5:00 pm. The flaw in the system was that it benefitted me greatly to get positive course review forms. Therefore, sometime between 3:00 – 3:30, I would pass out the course evaluations and tell the students that if they felt this class met all their needs, we could leave early. If not, we still had plenty of time to cover more material. The training center director would consistently tell me that I was the best teacher in the entire program. He had never seen such great reviews. Employee perception surveys can just as easily be manipulated.

The successful safety professional must define success for a safety program in the current organization at the current time. When defining success, be very careful to measure what needs to be measured. The number of accidents is greatly varied by pure luck. Most leading indicators only measure effort. Perception surveys only measure what the employees are motivated to tell management.

Constant improvement should be defined by a variety of factors. An important factor is the capacity of the organization to handle the obvious risks while having the capacity to handle the unexpected. When safety and operations are in sync, handling a crisis like COVID-19 becomes so much easier. Another factor of safety success is to measure how many resources are required to operate safely. Needing a large staff of nonworking safety inspectors to help make the organization operate safely is not a success. Spending more time, resources, and manpower on exclusively safety functions is sometimes measured as the organization's commitment to safety. The reality is that large expenditures of safety resources is a sign of band-aids covering safety failure. Safety success should be defined by great results without excessive resources being dedicated.

Takeaway 34: Adaptability must be built into the safety program.

Takeaway 35: Maintenance must be built into the safety program.

Takeaway 36: Constant improvement must be built into the safety program.

TAKEAWAYS

Takeaway 1: Focus on the process, not just the outcome.

Takeaway 2: Operational failures lead to safety failures.

Takeaway 3: Safety professionals can become too focused on Safety metrics alone.

Takeaway 4: Creating safety excellence must include operational excellence

Takeaway 5: Operational excellence cannot solely focus on production metrics

Takeaway 6: Safety professional must be just as concerned about Quality, Productivity, and Cost as other sectors should focus on Safety

Takeaway 7: Quantifying the Real Cost of Safety is Difficult

Takeaway 8: Quantifying the Actual Savings of Safety is Impossible

Takeaway 9: Accidents Happen Within Great Safety Programs

Takeaway 10: Compliance Is Only a Strategy of Safe Workplaces

Takeaway 11: Strategies Are Not the Goal

Takeaway 12: Focus on Compliance Limits Focus on Accident Prevention-Avoiding Hazards if possible, being aware of the highest risk activities

Takeaway 13: Honest and Open communication leads to better decisions

Takeaway 14: Clear expectations lead to success

Takeaway 15: Developing and Implementing an Action Plan is the First Step

Takeaway 16: Learn from Your Mistakes

Takeaway 17: Never Over Promise and Underdeliver

Takeaway 18: Be Your Own Worst Critic

Takeaway 19: Great Leaders needs Passion, Vision, and Problem Solving

Takeaway 20: In times of crisis, no job is more important than taking care of your team

Takeaway 21: Great Leadership emerges when problems are identified

Takeaway 22: Situational Bias based on past experiences

Takeaway 23: What's in it for me?

Takeaway 24: Assumptions lead both parties away from clear communication

Takeaway 25: Today's Construction safety professional can no longer be a compliance ambassador for OSHA.

Takeaway 26: Generational Differences create a need for different communication strategies Baby Boomers (born 1945-1964), Generations X (born 1965-1976), Y (Millennials-born 1977-1995), and Z (born after 1996.

Takeaway 27: The new normal will elevate the role of the safety professional in Commercial Construction.

Takeaway 28: Upon receiving information regarding a "Safety Violation," always seek out the facts and the circumstances before rushing to judgment and developing an action plan.

Takeaway 29: Occam's Razor, the simplest explanation for the problem is usually correct, but not always, there are exceptions.

Takeaway 30: Being correct does mean you will win. Winning is when all parties are satisfied with the option, and the situation at hand immediately improves.

Take Away 31: Changing Behaviors changes attitudes.

Take Away 32: Positive Reinforcement works,
Negative Reinforcement is rarely necessary.

Take Away 33: When Best Practices are
an expectation, Compliance is never even
mentioned.

Takeaway 34: Adaptability Must Be Built into the
Safety Program

Takeaway 35: Maintenance Must Be Built into
the Safety Program

Takeaway 36: Constant Improvement Must Be
Built into the Safety Program

www.ingramcontent.com/pod-product-compliance
Lightning Source LLC
Chambersburg PA
CBHW072202270326
41930CB00011B/2517